MIND DIET

COOKBOOK FOR

SENIORS OVER 70

100+ Quick and Nutritious Recipes Designed to Enhance Brain Health and Combat Memory Disorders.

Kingsley Klopp

Table of Contents

Poultry Recipes

Fish and Seafood Recipes

Vegetables

To show our appreciation for your purchase, we're delighted to offer you these special bonuses as a heartfelt thank you.

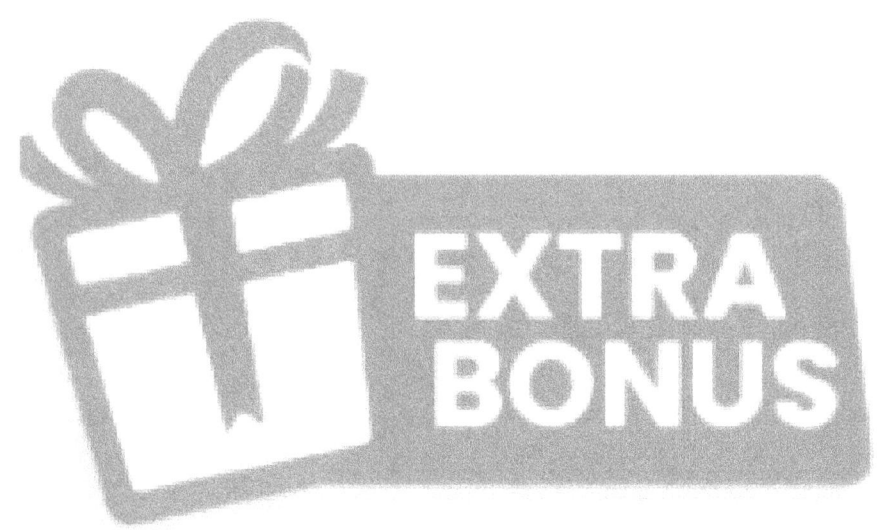

1. A Food Tracker Journal
2. Downloadable E-BOOK featuring full-color images of finished recipes

Important Note

We're excited to share this journey toward better brain health and delicious meals with you. As you explore these recipes, please remember that individual dietary needs can vary. It's important to adjust the recipes to suit your personal preferences and health requirements.

We encourage you to consult with your healthcare provider or a registered dietitian if you have any questions or concerns about how the MIND diet fits into your overall health plan. Your well-being is our priority, and professional guidance can help ensure that you're making the best choices for your unique situation.

Additionally, please note that the nutritional information provided is approximate and may vary based on the specific ingredients you use. Use this information as a general guide, and feel free to adapt as necessary.

Furthermore, If our cookbook has brought joy to your kitchen and table, we'd be thrilled to hear about your experiences in an Amazon review. On the flip side, if you stumble upon any hiccups while exploring our recipes, don't hesitate to get in touch at **kloppkingsley@gmail.com.** We're here to support your cooking journey every step of the way.

Introduction

Welcome to the journey of vibrant health and delicious eating! If you're holding this book, you're likely curious about how the MIND diet can transform your meals and, more importantly, your well-being. Let's set out on this journey together, exploring how mindful eating can boost brain health, enhance memory, and bring joy back to your kitchen.

The MIND diet, which stands for Mediterranean-DASH Intervention for Neurodegenerative Delay, is a combination of the Mediterranean and DASH diets. It's specifically designed to support brain health and reduce the risk of cognitive decline as we age. Packed with brain-boosting foods, the MIND diet emphasizes the importance of incorporating more leafy greens, berries, nuts, whole grains, and fish into your daily meals. You may be wondering why a cookbook specifically for seniors over 70. The answer is simple: as we age, our bodies and brains require different nutrients to function optimally. This cookbook is tailored to meet those unique needs, offering recipes that are not only delicious but also easy to prepare, considering any physical limitations you might face in the kitchen.

Imagine sitting down to a meal that not only tastes incredible but also supports your cognitive health. Picture savoring a vibrant berry salad, rich in antioxidants, or enjoying a warm bowl of whole grain oatmeal topped with fresh fruits and nuts. These aren't just meals; they're steps towards a healthier mind. Cooking shouldn't be a chore, especially at this stage of life. This cookbook is designed with simplicity in mind. We'll guide you through easy-to-follow recipes that don't require extensive culinary skills or fancy equipment. Each recipe is accompanied by clear instructions and tips to make preparation a breeze. Whether you're cooking for yourself or sharing meals with loved ones, these dishes are meant to be enjoyed without stress.

Eating well is one of the most enjoyable ways to take care of your brain and body. The MIND diet encourages a focus on whole, natural foods that are proven to support cognitive function. By incorporating more leafy greens, such as spinach and kale, and nutrient-dense foods like salmon and nuts, you're not only nourishing your body but also actively working to protect your brain. One of the great things about the MIND diet is its flexibility. We understand that dietary preferences and needs vary, and this cookbook offers a variety of options to suit your tastes. If you have dietary restrictions, we've included suggestions for substitutions and adaptations to ensure you can still enjoy the benefits of the MIND diet without feeling limited.

Change can be challenging, especially when it comes to altering eating habits. But remember, you're investing in your health and quality of life. Keep in mind the benefits: improved memory, enhanced cognitive function, and a potentially reduced risk of Alzheimer's disease. These are powerful motivators that can keep you committed to this new way of eating.

Now that you have an understanding of what the MIND diet is all about, it's time to dive into the recipes. From breakfast to dinner and everything in between, this cookbook offers a wide variety of meals that are sure to delight your taste buds and support your brain health. So grab your apron, and let's start cooking our way to a healthier, happier you!

Part 1: Understanding the MIND Diet
What is the MIND Diet?

The Mind Diet, which stands for the Mediterranean-DASH Intervention for Neurodegenerative Delay, is more than just a collection of foods; it's a powerful approach to eating that has the potential to transform your life, especially as you embrace your golden years. Imagine waking up every day feeling vibrant, with a mind as clear as a sunny morning. The Mind Diet is designed to make this a reality. It combines the best elements of two well-researched and highly respected diets—the Mediterranean diet and the DASH (Dietary Approaches to Stop Hypertension) diet—to create a nutritional plan specifically aimed at promoting brain health and reducing the risk of Alzheimer's disease and other forms of dementia.

The Essence of the Mind Diet

At its core, the Mind Diet emphasizes the consumption of ten brain-healthy food groups while limiting five unhealthy ones. It's not about strict rules or deprivation; it's about making delicious, nutritious choices that support your cognitive function and overall well-being.

Ten Brain-Healthy Food Groups:

1. Green Leafy Vegetables: Think of vibrant spinach, kale, and broccoli. These greens are packed with nutrients like vitamin K, folate, and beta-carotene, which have been shown to slow cognitive decline.
2. Other Vegetables: Variety is key. From colorful bell peppers to hearty carrots, each vegetable brings its own unique blend of vitamins, minerals, and antioxidants to the table.
3. Nuts: A handful of nuts each day can work wonders. Almonds, walnuts, and hazelnuts are rich in healthy fats, antioxidants, and vitamin E, all of which support brain health.
4. Berries: Bursting with flavor and antioxidants, berries like blueberries and strawberries help protect the brain from oxidative stress and inflammation.
5. Beans: These humble legumes are a powerhouse of protein, fiber, and nutrients. They help maintain steady blood sugar levels, providing sustained energy to the brain.
6. Whole Grains: Opt for whole wheat bread, oatmeal, and brown rice. Whole grains provide a steady release of glucose, the brain's primary energy source.
7. Fish: Especially fatty fish like salmon and sardines, which are rich in omega-3 fatty acids, crucial for brain health.
8. Poultry: Lean and versatile, poultry is a great source of protein and B vitamins, which support brain function.
9. Olive Oil: This golden elixir is the primary fat source in the Mediterranean diet, renowned for its anti-inflammatory properties.
10. Wine (in moderation): A glass of red wine with dinner can be part of the Mind Diet, thanks to its resveratrol content, which has been linked to brain health.

9. Olive Oil: This golden elixir is the primary fat source in the Mediterranean diet, renowned for its anti-inflammatory properties.

10. Wine (in moderation): A glass of red wine with dinner can be part of the Mind Diet, thanks to its resveratrol content, which has been linked to brain health.

Five Foods to Limit:

1. Red Meats: While a steak now and then is okay, try to limit your intake of red meats and opt for leaner protein sources more often.
2. Butter and Margarine: Use olive oil or other healthy fats instead.
3. Cheese: Delicious but best enjoyed in moderation.
4. Pastries and Sweets: These can be tempting but try to indulge only occasionally.
5. Fried or Fast Food: These foods are often high in unhealthy fats and should be limited.

The Science Behind the Mind Diet

In an age where cognitive decline and neurodegenerative diseases like Alzheimer's are on the rise, the search for effective preventive measures has never been more urgent. The Mind Diet, standing for the Mediterranean-DASH Intervention for Neurodegenerative Delay, offers a beacon of hope, combining the most beneficial elements of the Mediterranean diet and the DASH (Dietary Approaches to Stop Hypertension) diet. This innovative dietary approach is designed to nourish the brain, and its effectiveness is backed by compelling scientific research.

The Foundation of the Mind Diet

The Mind Diet is built upon two well-established diets:

1. The Mediterranean Diet: Originating from the eating habits of people in Mediterranean countries, this diet emphasizes fruits, vegetables, whole grains, nuts, and olive oil, with moderate consumption of fish and poultry, and limited intake of red meat and sweets.
2. The DASH Diet: Developed to combat high blood pressure, the DASH diet focuses on fruits, vegetables, whole grains, lean proteins, and low-fat dairy, while reducing salt, red meat, and sugar-sweetened foods and beverages.

The Mind Diet integrates these principles to specifically target brain health. It emphasizes ten brain-healthy food groups while limiting five unhealthy ones. These dietary choices are rooted in the latest scientific understanding of how nutrients affect cognitive function and neurodegeneration.

The Role of Antioxidants and Anti-inflammatory Compounds

A central premise of the Mind Diet is its focus on foods rich in antioxidants and anti-inflammatory compounds. These substances combat oxidative stress and inflammation, two major contributors to cognitive decline and neurodegenerative diseases.

Oxidative Stress: This occurs when there is an imbalance between free radicals (unstable molecules that can damage cells) and antioxidants in the body. Free radicals are generated through normal metabolic processes and external factors like pollution and radiation. Antioxidants neutralize free radicals, preventing cell damage. Foods such as berries, leafy greens, and nuts are rich in antioxidants like vitamins C and E, flavonoids, and carotenoids, which help protect brain cells from oxidative stress.

Inflammation: Chronic inflammation in the brain is a hallmark of neurodegenerative diseases. The Mind Diet includes foods with anti-inflammatory properties, such as fatty fish rich in omega-3 fatty acids, olive oil, and nuts. Omega-3s, particularly DHA (docosahexaenoic acid), are crucial for maintaining the structural integrity of brain cells and reducing inflammation.

The Impact of Specific Nutrients on Brain Health

Several key nutrients in the Mind Diet play vital roles in brain function and protection against cognitive decline:

1. Omega-3 Fatty Acids: Found in fatty fish (e.g., salmon, sardines), flaxseeds, and walnuts, omega-3s are essential for maintaining cell membrane integrity in the brain. They also promote the production of anti-inflammatory molecules and have been shown to enhance synaptic plasticity, which is crucial for learning and memory.

2. B Vitamins: Foods like leafy greens, legumes, and whole grains are rich in B vitamins, particularly folate, B6, and B12. These vitamins are essential for reducing homocysteine levels, an amino acid associated with increased risk of cognitive decline and Alzheimer's disease when elevated.

3. Vitamin E: Nuts and seeds, such as almonds and sunflower seeds, are excellent sources of vitamin E, an antioxidant that protects brain cells from oxidative damage. Higher intake of vitamin E has been linked to slower cognitive decline in elderly individuals.

4. Polyphenols: Berries, red wine (in moderation), and olive oil are rich in polyphenols, which are potent antioxidants with anti-inflammatory properties. Polyphenols have been shown to improve cognitive function and protect against age-related cognitive decline.

Scientific Evidence Supporting the Mind Diet

The effectiveness of the Mind Diet is supported by rigorous scientific research. A landmark study conducted by researchers at Rush University Medical Center in Chicago followed nearly 1,000 elderly individuals over a period of up to 10 years. The study found that those who closely adhered to the Mind Diet had a 53% reduced risk of developing Alzheimer's disease compared to those who did not follow the diet. Even moderate adherence to the diet was associated with a 35% reduction in risk.

Moreover, individuals following the Mind Diet consistently scored higher on cognitive tests over time. This suggests that the diet not only reduces the risk of cognitive decline but also helps maintain cognitive function in older adults.

Another study published in the journal "Alzheimer's & Dementia" found that the Mind Diet was associated with slower rates of cognitive decline among participants. This research underscores the potential of dietary interventions to preserve brain health and delay the onset of neurodegenerative diseases.

How the Mind Diet Promotes Brain Health

The Synergy of Nutrient-Rich Foods

The Mind Diet emphasizes the consumption of ten brain-healthy food groups while limiting five unhealthy ones. This balanced approach ensures that the brain receives an optimal mix of nutrients, antioxidants, and anti-inflammatory compounds.

Green Leafy Vegetables: Spinach, kale, and other leafy greens are rich in vitamins A and C, which are powerful antioxidants. These vitamins help reduce oxidative stress, a key factor in the aging of brain cells. Regular consumption of these vegetables has been linked to slower cognitive decline.

Other Vegetables: A variety of vegetables provides a wide range of nutrients essential for brain health. For example, bell peppers and carrots are high in beta-carotene, a precursor to vitamin A, which supports vision and cognitive function.

Nuts: Almonds, walnuts, and other nuts are packed with healthy fats, vitamin E, and antioxidants. Vitamin E, in particular, is known for its role in protecting brain cells from oxidative damage. Studies have shown that higher intake of vitamin E is associated with better cognitive performance in older adults.

Berries: Blueberries, strawberries, and other berries are rich in flavonoids, which are potent antioxidants. Flavonoids help improve memory and cognitive function by enhancing brain cell signaling and reducing inflammation.

Beans: Legumes such as lentils and chickpeas are excellent sources of protein, fiber, and B vitamins. B vitamins, particularly folate, B6, and B12, are crucial for brain health as they help reduce homocysteine levels, which are associated with cognitive decline.

Whole Grains: Whole grains like oatmeal, brown rice, and whole wheat bread provide a steady supply of glucose, the brain's primary energy source. They also contain fiber, which supports overall health and prevents spikes in blood sugar levels.

Fish: Fatty fish such as salmon and sardines are rich in omega-3 fatty acids, particularly DHA (docosahexaenoic acid), which is essential for maintaining the structure and function of brain cells. Omega-3s also have anti-inflammatory properties that help protect the brain from damage.

Poultry: Chicken and turkey are lean sources of protein and B vitamins. These nutrients are vital for neurotransmitter production and brain function.

Olive Oil: Olive oil is a staple of the Mediterranean diet and is known for its anti-inflammatory and antioxidant properties. The polyphenols in olive oil help protect the brain from oxidative stress and inflammation.

Wine (in moderation): Red wine, consumed in moderation, is rich in resveratrol, a compound that has been shown to protect brain cells from damage and improve blood flow to the brain.

Mechanisms of Brain Protection

1. Reducing Oxidative Stress: Oxidative stress occurs when there is an imbalance between free radicals and antioxidants in the body. Free radicals can damage brain cells and contribute to cognitive decline. The Mind Diet includes a variety of antioxidant-rich foods, such as berries, nuts, and green leafy vegetables, which help neutralize free radicals and protect brain cells from damage.

2. Anti-inflammatory Effects: Chronic inflammation is a major contributor to neurodegenerative diseases like Alzheimer's. The Mind Diet emphasizes foods with anti-inflammatory properties, such as fatty fish, olive oil, and nuts. Omega-3 fatty acids in fish and polyphenols in olive oil help reduce inflammation in the brain, protecting it from damage.

3. Supporting Neurogenesis and Synaptic Plasticity: Neurogenesis is the process of forming new neurons, while synaptic plasticity refers to the ability of synapses (the connections between neurons) to strengthen or weaken over time. Both processes are essential for learning, memory, and overall cognitive function. The nutrients in the Mind Diet, particularly omega-3 fatty acids, B vitamins, and antioxidants, support neurogenesis and synaptic plasticity, enhancing cognitive abilities.

4. Enhancing Blood Flow to the Brain: Good blood flow is crucial for delivering oxygen and nutrients to brain cells. The Mind Diet promotes cardiovascular health through its emphasis on heart-healthy foods like whole grains, fish, and olive oil. Improved cardiovascular health translates to better blood flow to the brain, which supports cognitive function.

5. Regulating Blood Sugar Levels: Fluctuations in blood sugar levels can affect brain function. The Mind Diet includes complex carbohydrates from whole grains, which provide a steady release of glucose to the brain. This helps maintain stable blood sugar levels, ensuring a consistent supply of energy to the brain.

Scientific Evidence and Research: Numerous studies support the effectiveness of the Mind Diet in promoting brain health. For instance, research conducted by Rush University Medical Center found that adherence to the Mind Diet was associated with a significantly lower risk of Alzheimer's disease. Participants who closely followed the diet had a 53% reduced risk, while even moderate adherence resulted in a 35% reduction.

Another study published in the journal "Alzheimer's & Dementia" showed that the Mind Diet slowed cognitive decline among older adults, highlighting its potential to preserve brain function over time.

Benefits of the Mind Diet for Seniors

As we age, maintaining cognitive health and overall well-being becomes increasingly important. The Mind Diet, which stands for the Mediterranean-DASH Intervention for Neurodegenerative Delay, offers a unique and scientifically-backed approach to nutrition that specifically targets brain health. Designed to slow cognitive decline and reduce the risk of Alzheimer's disease, the Mind Diet combines elements of the Mediterranean diet and the DASH diet. For seniors, the benefits of adopting the Mind Diet are profound and far-reaching, impacting not only brain health but also overall physical and emotional well-being.

1. Slows Cognitive Decline
One of the most compelling benefits of the Mind Diet is its potential to slow cognitive decline. Studies have shown that adhering to the Mind Diet can significantly reduce the risk of Alzheimer's disease and other forms of dementia. By focusing on brain-healthy foods rich in antioxidants, anti-inflammatory compounds, and essential nutrients, the Mind Diet helps protect brain cells from damage and supports cognitive function.
Scientific Evidence: Research conducted by Rush University Medical Center found that seniors who followed the Mind Diet closely had a 53% reduced risk of Alzheimer's disease. Even moderate adherence to the diet resulted in a 35% reduction in risk. This demonstrates the powerful impact that dietary choices can have on cognitive health.

2. Enhances Memory and Learning
The nutrients emphasized in the Mind Diet, such as omega-3 fatty acids, B vitamins, and antioxidants, play crucial roles in supporting memory and learning. Omega-3 fatty acids, found in fatty fish like salmon and sardines, are essential for maintaining the structure and function of brain cells. B vitamins, particularly folate, B6, and B12, help reduce homocysteine levels, which are associated with cognitive decline.
Mechanisms: These nutrients support neurogenesis (the formation of new neurons) and synaptic plasticity (the ability of synapses to strengthen or weaken over time), both of which are essential for learning and memory. By enhancing these processes, the Mind Diet helps seniors maintain and improve their cognitive abilities.

3. Reduces Inflammation
Chronic inflammation is a major contributor to cognitive decline and neurodegenerative diseases. The Mind Diet includes foods with potent anti-inflammatory properties, such as fatty fish, olive oil, nuts, and leafy greens. Omega-3 fatty acids in fish and polyphenols in olive oil help reduce inflammation in the brain, protecting it from damage.
Impact on Brain Health: By reducing inflammation, the Mind Diet helps protect brain cells from the harmful effects of chronic inflammation, thereby preserving cognitive function and reducing the risk of neurodegenerative diseases.

4. Supports Heart Health

Good cardiovascular health is essential for maintaining cognitive function, as the brain relies on a steady supply of oxygen and nutrients delivered through the bloodstream. The Mind Diet promotes heart health by emphasizing heart-healthy foods such as whole grains, fish, olive oil, and nuts, while limiting red meat, butter, and sweets.

Heart-Brain Connection: Improved cardiovascular health leads to better blood flow to the brain, ensuring that brain cells receive the oxygen and nutrients they need to function optimally. This, in turn, supports cognitive health and reduces the risk of stroke and other cardiovascular-related cognitive impairments.

5. Stabilizes Blood Sugar Levels

Fluctuations in blood sugar levels can negatively impact brain function. The Mind Diet includes complex carbohydrates from whole grains, vegetables, and legumes, which provide a steady release of glucose to the brain. This helps maintain stable blood sugar levels, ensuring a consistent supply of energy to the brain.

Benefits for Cognitive Function: Stable blood sugar levels prevent the cognitive impairment associated with high and low blood sugar spikes, supporting overall brain health and cognitive function.

6. Promotes Overall Physical Health

Beyond its cognitive benefits, the Mind Diet also supports overall physical health. The diet's emphasis on whole, nutrient-dense foods helps seniors maintain a healthy weight, reduce the risk of chronic diseases such as diabetes and hypertension, and improve their overall quality of life.

Nutrient-Rich Foods: The variety of fruits, vegetables, whole grains, nuts, and lean proteins in the Mind Diet provides essential vitamins, minerals, and other nutrients that support overall health and well-being.

7. Improves Mood and Emotional Well-being

Nutrition plays a crucial role in mental health. The Mind Diet, rich in omega-3 fatty acids, antioxidants, and other essential nutrients, has been linked to improved mood and emotional well-being. Omega-3s, in particular, have been shown to reduce symptoms of depression and anxiety.

Psychological Benefits: By supporting brain health and reducing inflammation, the Mind Diet helps improve mood, reduce stress, and enhance overall emotional well-being, contributing to a better quality of life for seniors.

8. Increases Longevity

Adopting the Mind Diet can contribute to increased longevity. The diet's emphasis on heart-healthy, anti-inflammatory, and nutrient-dense foods supports overall health, reduces the risk of chronic diseases, and promotes a longer, healthier life.

Longevity Studies: Research has shown that diets similar to the Mind Diet, such as the Mediterranean diet, are associated with increased longevity and a lower risk of mortality from all causes.

Breakfast Recipes

1. Oatmeal with Blueberries
Ingredients:
- 1 cup rolled oats
- 2 cups water or unsweetened almond milk
- 1 cup fresh blueberries
- 1 tablespoon chia seeds
- 1 teaspoon ground cinnamon
- 1 tablespoon honey or maple syrup (optional)
- 1/4 cup chopped walnuts

Instructions:
1. In a medium saucepan, bring the water or almond milk to a boil.
2. Add the rolled oats and reduce the heat to medium-low. Cook, stirring occasionally, for about 5 minutes or until the oats are tender and the liquid is absorbed.
3. Stir in the ground cinnamon and chia seeds.
4. Remove from heat and let the oatmeal sit for a minute.
5. Serve the oatmeal in bowls, topped with fresh blueberries and chopped walnuts.
6. Drizzle with honey or maple syrup if desired.

Nutrition Info per Serving (Serves 2):
- Calories: 350
- Protein: 9g
- Carbohydrates: 55g
- Dietary Fiber: 10g
- Sugars: 13g
- Total Fat: 12g
- Saturated Fat: 1g
- Sodium: 10mg

Servings: 2 Cooking Time: 10 minutes

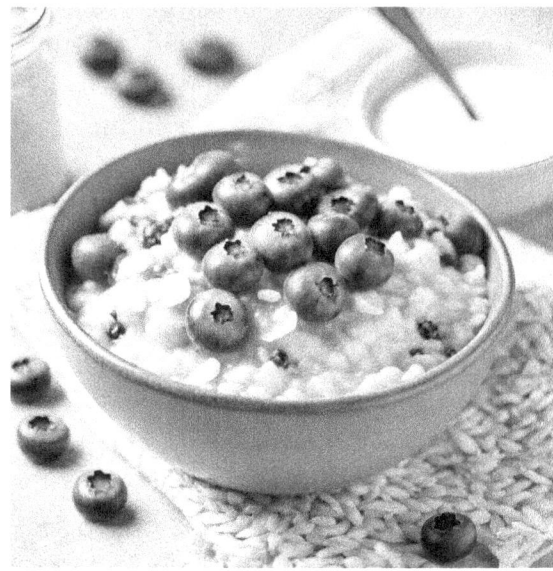

2. Spinach and Feta Omelette

Ingredients:

- 4 large eggs
- 1/4 cup unsweetened almond milk
- 1 cup fresh spinach, chopped
- 1/4 cup crumbled feta cheese
- 1 tablespoon olive oil
- 1/4 teaspoon garlic powder
- 1/4 teaspoon onion powder
- Freshly ground black pepper, to taste

Instructions:

1. In a medium bowl, whisk together the eggs, almond milk, garlic powder, onion powder, and black pepper.
2. Heat olive oil in a non-stick skillet over medium heat.
3. Add the chopped spinach and cook until wilted, about 2 minutes.
4. Pour the egg mixture into the skillet over the spinach. Cook without stirring for about 3 minutes, or until the edges start to set.
5. Sprinkle the crumbled feta cheese evenly over one half of the omelette.
6. Using a spatula, fold the omelette in half and cook for another 2 minutes, or until the eggs are fully set and the cheese is melted.
7. Slide the omelette onto a plate and serve immediately.

Nutrition Info per Serving (Serves 2):

- Calories: 220
- Protein: 14g
- Carbohydrates: 3g
- Dietary Fiber: 1g
- Sugars: 1g
- Total Fat: 18g
- Saturated Fat: 6g
- Sodium: 320mg

Servings: 2 Cooking Time: 10 minutes

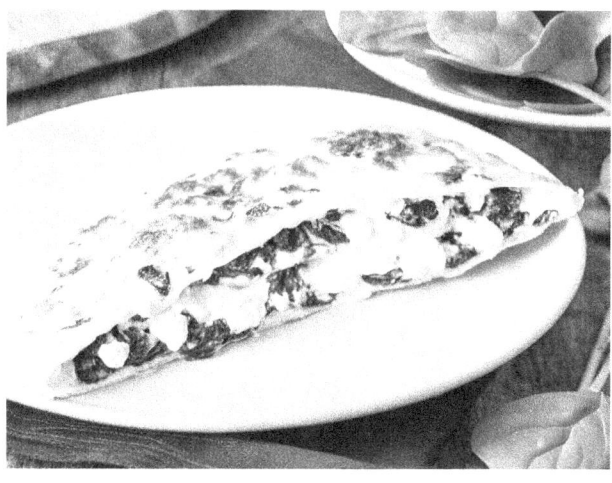

3. Greek Yogurt Parfait

Ingredients:

- 2 cups plain Greek yogurt
- 1 cup mixed fresh berries (strawberries, blueberries, raspberries)
- 1/4 cup granola (low-sugar, whole grain)
- 2 tablespoons honey
- 1 tablespoon chia seeds

Instructions:

1. In a bowl, mix the Greek yogurt with honey until well combined.
2. In serving glasses or bowls, layer half of the yogurt at the bottom.
3. Add a layer of mixed berries.
4. Sprinkle with chia seeds and granola.
5. Repeat the layers with the remaining yogurt, berries, chia seeds, and granola.
6. Serve immediately or refrigerate until ready to serve.

Nutrition Info per Serving (Serves 2):

- Calories: 250
- Protein: 15g
- Carbohydrates: 35g
- Dietary Fiber: 5g
- Sugars: 20g
- Total Fat: 6g
- Saturated Fat: 2g
- Sodium: 60mg

Servings: 2 Cooking Time: 5 minutes

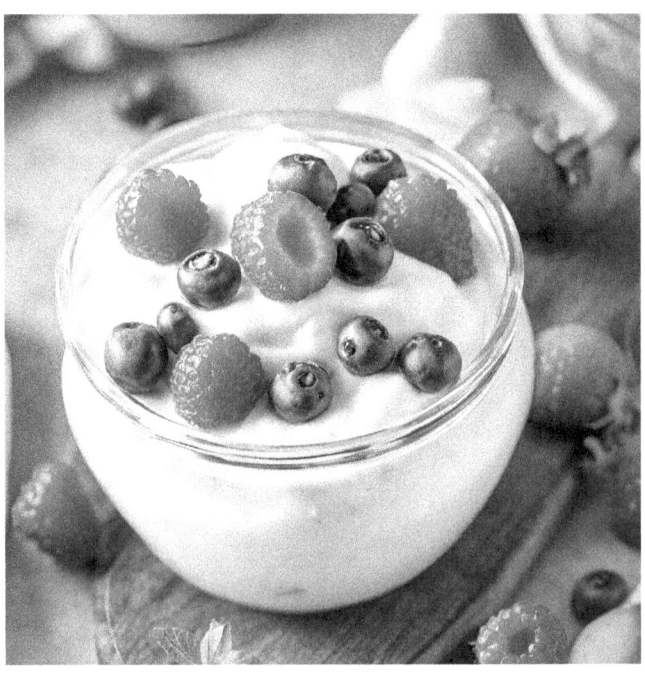

4. Whole Grain Pancakes

Ingredients:

- 1 cup whole wheat flour
- 1 tablespoon baking powder
- 1 tablespoon ground flaxseed
- 1 cup unsweetened almond milk
- 1 large egg
- 2 tablespoons olive oil
- 1 teaspoon vanilla extract
- 1 tablespoon honey or maple syrup
- 1/2 cup fresh blueberries (optional)

Instructions:

1. In a large bowl, whisk together the whole wheat flour, baking powder, and ground flaxseed.
2. In another bowl, whisk together the almond milk, egg, olive oil, vanilla extract, and honey or maple syrup.
3. Pour the wet ingredients into the dry ingredients and stir until just combined. Do not overmix. Fold in the blueberries if using.
4. Heat a non-stick skillet or griddle over medium heat and lightly grease with olive oil.
5. Pour 1/4 cup of batter onto the skillet for each pancake. Cook until bubbles form on the surface, then flip and cook until golden brown, about 2 minutes per side.
6. Serve the pancakes warm with additional blueberries and a drizzle of honey or maple syrup if desired.

Nutrition Info per Serving (Serves 4):

- Calories: 180
- Protein: 5g
- Carbohydrates: 26g
- Dietary Fiber: 4g
- Sugars: 8g
- Total Fat: 7g
- Saturated Fat: 1g
- Sodium: 230mg

Servings: 4 Cooking Time: 20 minutes

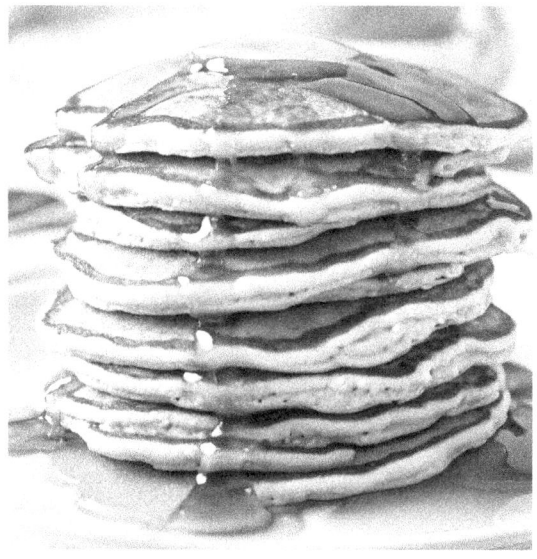

5. Quinoa Porridge

Ingredients:

- 1 cup quinoa, rinsed
- 2 cups unsweetened almond milk
- 1 tablespoon chia seeds
- 1 teaspoon ground cinnamon
- 1 tablespoon honey or maple syrup
- 1/2 cup fresh berries (blueberries, strawberries, or raspberries)
- 1/4 cup chopped almonds

Instructions:

1. In a medium saucepan, bring the quinoa and almond milk to a boil.
2. Reduce the heat to low, cover, and simmer for about 15 minutes or until the quinoa is tender and the liquid is absorbed.
3. Stir in the chia seeds, ground cinnamon, and honey or maple syrup.
4. Serve the porridge in bowls, topped with fresh berries and chopped almonds.

Nutrition Info per Serving (Serves 2):

- Calories: 350
- Protein: 10g
- Carbohydrates: 55g
- Dietary Fiber: 8g
- Sugars: 14g
- Total Fat: 12g
- Saturated Fat: 1g
- Sodium: 40mg

Servings: 2 Cooking Time: 20 minutes

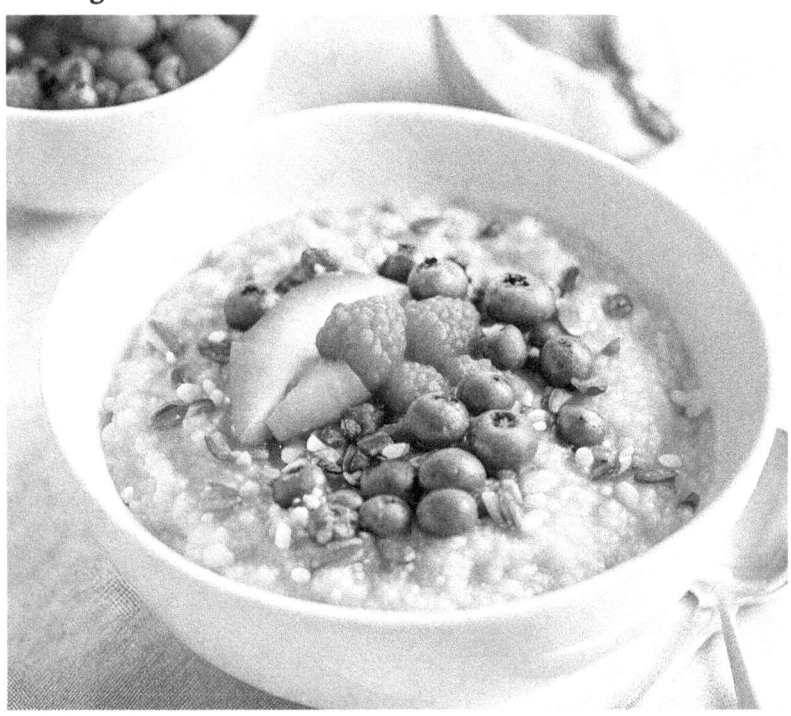

6. Turkey Sausage and Veggie Hash

Ingredients:

- 1 tablespoon olive oil
- 1 cup diced sweet potato
- 1/2 cup diced red bell pepper
- 1/2 cup diced zucchini
- 1/2 cup chopped onion
- 2 cloves garlic, minced
- 1 cup cooked turkey sausage, crumbled
- 1 teaspoon paprika
- 1 teaspoon dried oregano
- Freshly ground black pepper, to taste

Instructions:

1. Heat olive oil in a large skillet over medium heat.
2. Add the diced sweet potato and cook for 5-7 minutes until slightly tender.
3. Add the red bell pepper, zucchini, and onion, and cook for another 5 minutes until vegetables are tender.
4. Stir in the minced garlic and cook for 1 minute until fragrant.
5. Add the cooked turkey sausage, paprika, dried oregano, and black pepper, and cook for 3-4 minutes until heated through.
6. Serve the hash warm.

Nutrition Info per Serving (Serves 4):

- Calories: 210
- Protein: 14g
- Carbohydrates: 20g
- Dietary Fiber: 4g
- Sugars: 6g
- Total Fat: 9g
- Saturated Fat: 2g
- Sodium: 300mg

Servings: 4 Cooking Time: 20 minutes

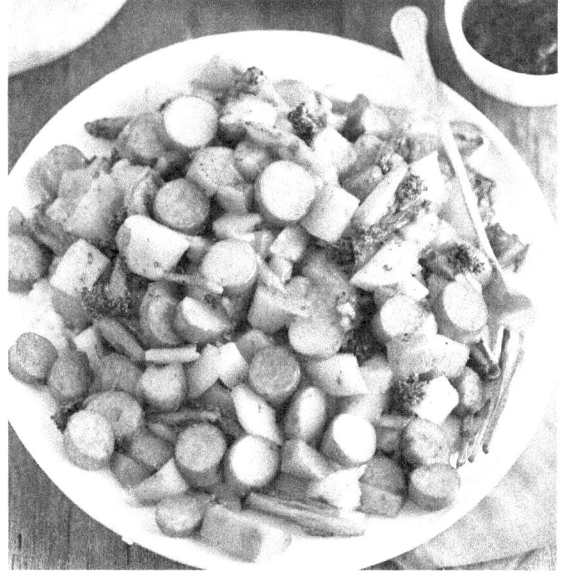

7. Mushroom and Spinach Frittata

Ingredients:

- 6 large eggs
- 1/4 cup unsweetened almond milk
- 1 tablespoon olive oil
- 1 cup sliced mushrooms
- 1 cup fresh spinach, chopped
- 1/4 cup crumbled feta cheese
- 1 teaspoon garlic powder
- Freshly ground black pepper, to taste

Instructions:

1. Preheat the oven to 375°F (190°C).
2. In a bowl, whisk together the eggs, almond milk, garlic powder, and black pepper.
3. Heat olive oil in an oven-safe skillet over medium heat.
4. Add the sliced mushrooms and cook for 3-4 minutes until tender.
5. Add the chopped spinach and cook until wilted, about 2 minutes.
6. Pour the egg mixture over the vegetables and sprinkle with crumbled feta cheese.
7. Transfer the skillet to the oven and bake for 15-20 minutes, or until the eggs are set.
8. Slice and serve the frittata warm.

Nutrition Info per Serving (Serves 4):

- Calories: 180
- Protein: 12g
- Carbohydrates: 3g
- Dietary Fiber: 1g
- Sugars: 1g
- Total Fat: 14g
- Saturated Fat: 5g
- Sodium: 270mg

Servings: 4 Cooking Time: 25 minutes

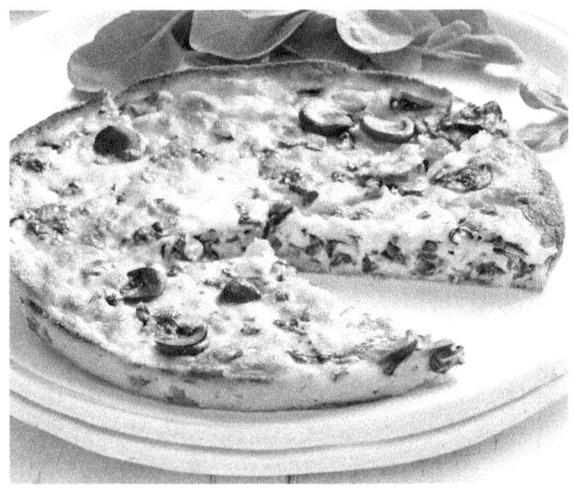

8. Almond Butter Banana Toast

Ingredients:

- 4 slices whole grain bread
- 4 tablespoons almond butter
- 2 ripe bananas, sliced
- 1 tablespoon chia seeds
- 1 teaspoon ground cinnamon

Instructions:

1. Toast the whole grain bread slices until golden brown.
2. Spread 1 tablespoon of almond butter on each slice of toast.
3. Top each slice with banana slices.
4. Sprinkle with chia seeds and ground cinnamon.
5. Serve immediately.

Nutrition Info per Serving (Serves 4):

- Calories: 250
- Protein: 7g
- Carbohydrates: 40g
- Dietary Fiber: 7g
- Sugars: 12g
- Total Fat: 9g
- Saturated Fat: 1g
- Sodium: 140mg

Servings: 4 Cooking Time: 5 minutes

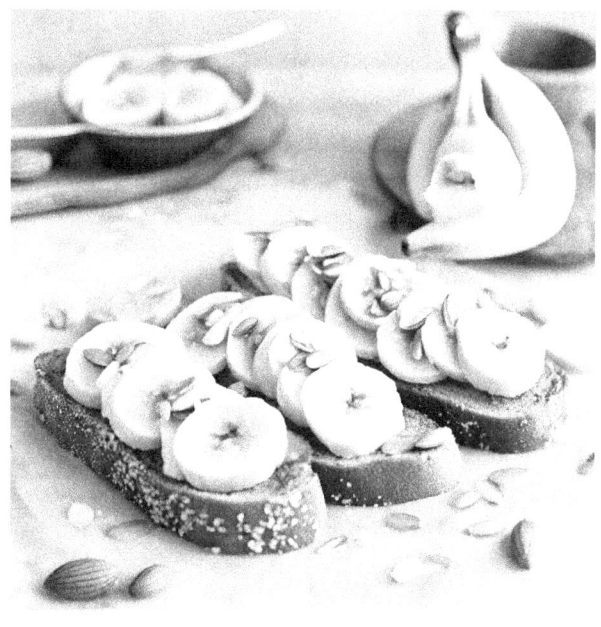

9. Kale and Tomato Quiche

Ingredients:

- 1 prepared whole grain pie crust
- 1 tablespoon olive oil
- 1 cup chopped kale
- 1 cup cherry tomatoes, halved
- 1/2 cup crumbled feta cheese
- 6 large eggs
- 1/2 cup unsweetened almond milk
- 1 teaspoon dried basil
- Freshly ground black pepper, to taste

Instructions:

1. Preheat the oven to 375°F (190°C).
2. Heat olive oil in a skillet over medium heat.
3. Add the chopped kale and cook until wilted, about 3 minutes.
4. In a bowl, whisk together the eggs, almond milk, dried basil, and black pepper.
5. Spread the wilted kale, cherry tomatoes, and crumbled feta cheese evenly over the pie crust.
6. Pour the egg mixture over the vegetables and cheese.
7. Bake for 30-35 minutes, or until the quiche is set and golden brown on top.
8. Let the quiche cool for a few minutes before slicing and serving.

Nutrition Info per Serving (Serves 6):

- Calories: 220
- Protein: 10g
- Carbohydrates: 15g
- Dietary Fiber: 2g
- Sugars: 3g
- Total Fat: 13g
- Saturated Fat: 4g
- Sodium: 260mg

Servings: 6 Cooking Time: 45 minutes

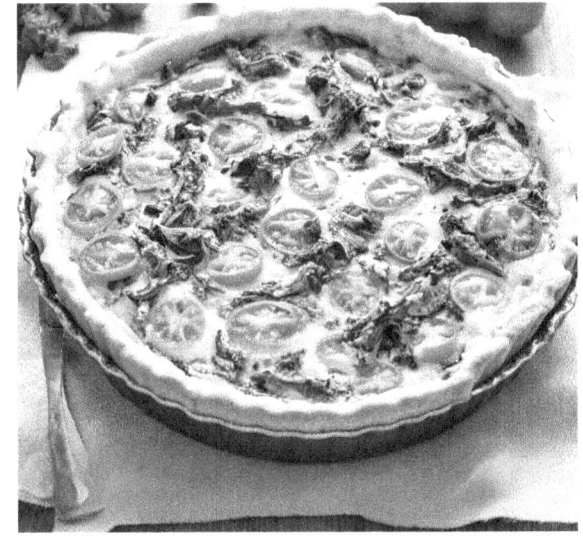

10. Berry and Walnut Oatmeal

Ingredients:

- 1 cup rolled oats
- 2 cups water or unsweetened almond milk
- 1 cup mixed berries (blueberries, strawberries, raspberries)
- 1/4 cup chopped walnuts
- 1 tablespoon chia seeds
- 1 teaspoon ground cinnamon
- 1 tablespoon honey or maple syrup (optional)

Instructions:

1. In a medium saucepan, bring the water or almond milk to a boil.
2. Add the rolled oats and reduce the heat to medium-low. Cook, stirring occasionally, for about 5 minutes or until the oats are tender and the liquid is absorbed.
3. Stir in the ground cinnamon and chia seeds.
4. Remove from heat and let the oatmeal sit for a minute.
5. Serve the oatmeal in bowls, topped with mixed berries and chopped walnuts.
6. Drizzle with honey or maple syrup if desired.

Nutrition Info per Serving (Serves 2):

- Calories: 320
- Protein: 8g
- Carbohydrates: 50g
- Dietary Fiber: 8g
- Sugars: 12g
- Total Fat: 11g
- Saturated Fat: 1g
- Sodium: 10mg

Servings: 2 Cooking Time: 10 minutes

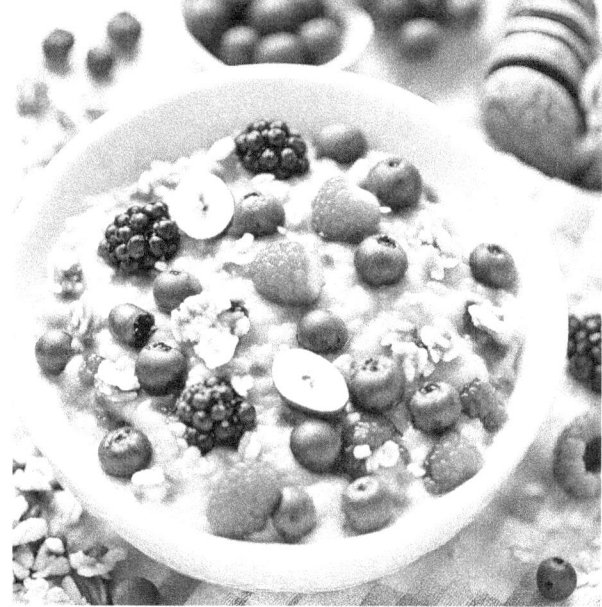

11. Vegetable Muffins

Ingredients:

- 1 cup whole wheat flour
- 1/2 cup rolled oats
- 1 teaspoon baking powder
- 1/2 teaspoon baking soda
- 1 teaspoon garlic powder
- 1 teaspoon onion powder
- 1/2 cup grated zucchini
- 1/2 cup grated carrot
- 1/2 cup chopped spinach
- 1/4 cup crumbled feta cheese
- 2 large eggs
- 1/2 cup unsweetened almond milk
- 1/4 cup olive oil
- 1 teaspoon dried oregano

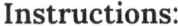

Instructions:

1. Preheat the oven to 375°F (190°C) and line a muffin tin with paper liners.
2. In a large bowl, whisk together the whole wheat flour, rolled oats, baking powder, baking soda, garlic powder, onion powder, and dried oregano.
3. In another bowl, whisk together the eggs, almond milk, and olive oil.
4. Add the wet ingredients to the dry ingredients and stir until just combined.
5. Fold in the grated zucchini, grated carrot, chopped spinach, and crumbled feta cheese.
6. Divide the batter evenly among the muffin cups.
7. Bake for 20-25 minutes, or until a toothpick inserted into the center comes out clean.
8. Let the muffins cool in the tin for a few minutes before transferring to a wire rack to cool completely.

Nutrition Info per Serving (Serves 12):

- Calories: 120
- Protein: 4g
- Carbohydrates: 12g
- Dietary Fiber: 2g
- Sugars: 2g
- Total Fat: 7g
- Saturated Fat: 1g
- Sodium: 100mg

Servings: 12 muffins Cooking Time: 30 minutes

12. Pumpkin Spice Smoothie

Ingredients:

- 1 cup unsweetened almond milk
- 1/2 cup canned pumpkin puree
- 1 frozen banana
- 1 tablespoon chia seeds
- 1 teaspoon ground cinnamon
- 1/4 teaspoon ground nutmeg
- 1/4 teaspoon ground ginger
- 1 tablespoon honey or maple syrup (optional)

Instructions:

1. In a blender, combine the almond milk, pumpkin puree, frozen banana, chia seeds, ground cinnamon, ground nutmeg, and ground ginger.
2. Blend until smooth.
3. Taste and add honey or maple syrup if desired for additional sweetness.
4. Pour into a glass and serve immediately.

Nutrition Info per Serving (Serves 1):

- Calories: 200
- Protein: 4g
- Carbohydrates: 42g
- Dietary Fiber: 8g
- Sugars: 21g
- Total Fat: 4g
- Saturated Fat: 0.5g
- Sodium: 100mg

Servings: 1 Cooking Time: 5 minutes

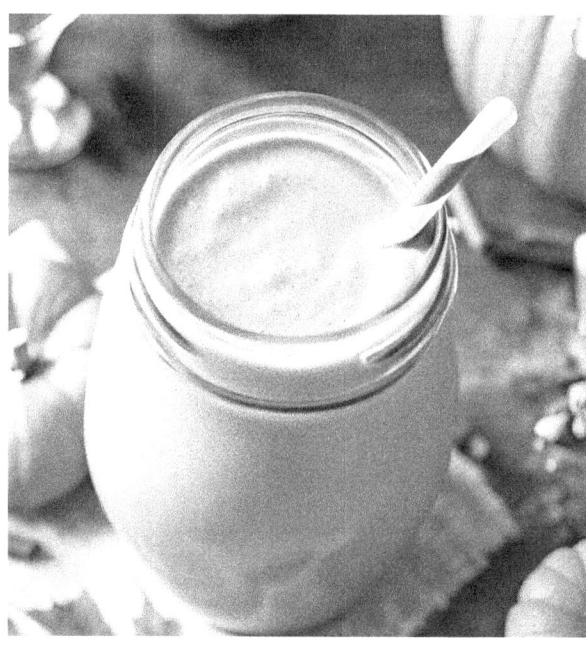

13. Broccoli and Cheese Omelette

Ingredients:

- 4 large eggs
- 1/4 cup unsweetened almond milk
- 1 cup steamed broccoli florets, chopped
- 1/4 cup crumbled feta cheese
- 1 tablespoon olive oil
- 1/2 teaspoon garlic powder
- Freshly ground black pepper, to taste

Instructions:

1. In a medium bowl, whisk together the eggs, almond milk, garlic powder, and black pepper.
2. Heat olive oil in a non-stick skillet over medium heat.
3. Pour the egg mixture into the skillet and cook without stirring for about 3 minutes, or until the edges start to set.
4. Sprinkle the chopped broccoli and crumbled feta cheese evenly over one half of the omelette.
5. Using a spatula, fold the omelette in half and cook for another 2 minutes, or until the eggs are fully set and the cheese is melted.
6. Slide the omelette onto a plate and serve immediately.

Nutrition Info per Serving (Serves 2):

- Calories: 210
- Protein: 14g
- Carbohydrates: 5g
- Dietary Fiber: 2g
- Sugars: 1g
- Total Fat: 15g
- Saturated Fat: 5g
- Sodium: 300mg

Servings: 2 Cooking Time: 10 minutes

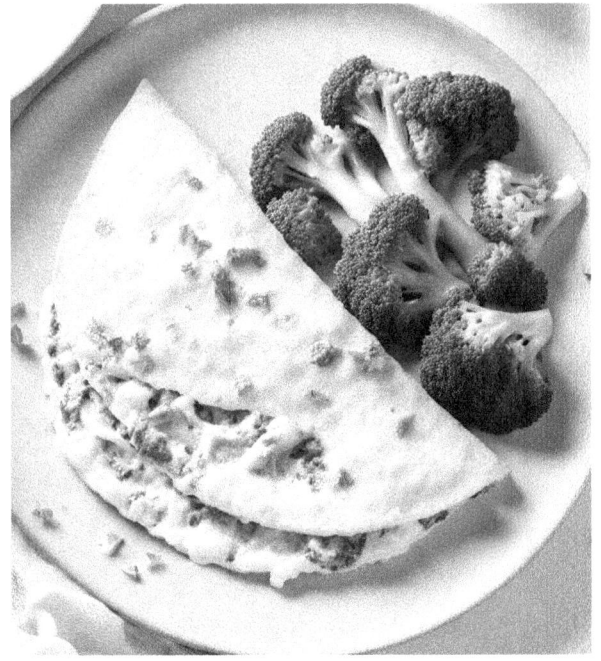

14. Sweet Potato and Kale Bowl

Ingredients:

- 1 large sweet potato, peeled and diced
- 2 tablespoons olive oil, divided
- 2 cups chopped kale, stems removed
- 1/2 cup cooked quinoa
- 1/4 cup chopped walnuts
- 1 tablespoon balsamic vinegar
- 1/2 teaspoon garlic powder
- 1/2 teaspoon onion powder
- Freshly ground black pepper, to taste

Instructions:

1. Preheat the oven to 400°F (200°C).
2. Toss the diced sweet potato with 1 tablespoon of olive oil, garlic powder, and onion powder. Spread on a baking sheet and roast for 20-25 minutes, or until tender and lightly browned.
3. While the sweet potato is roasting, heat the remaining olive oil in a large skillet over medium heat.
4. Add the chopped kale and cook until wilted, about 5 minutes.
5. In a bowl, combine the roasted sweet potato, cooked quinoa, and wilted kale.
6. Drizzle with balsamic vinegar and sprinkle with chopped walnuts.
7. Toss to combine and serve warm.

Nutrition Info per Serving (Serves 2):

- Calories: 300
- Protein: 7g
- Carbohydrates: 40g
- Dietary Fiber: 7g
- Sugars: 8g
- Total Fat: 14g
- Saturated Fat: 2g
- Sodium: 60mg

Servings: 2 Cooking Time: 30 minutes

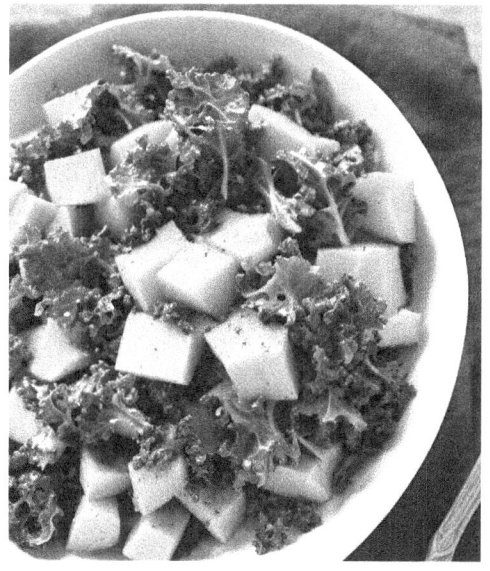

15. Apple Cinnamon Steel-Cut Oats

Ingredients:

- 1 cup steel-cut oats
- 4 cups water
- 1 apple, peeled, cored, and diced
- 1 teaspoon ground cinnamon
- 1 tablespoon chia seeds
- 1 tablespoon honey or maple syrup (optional)
- 1/4 cup chopped walnuts

Instructions:

1. In a medium saucepan, bring the water to a boil.
2. Add the steel-cut oats, reduce the heat to low, and simmer for about 20-25 minutes, stirring occasionally, until the oats are tender.
3. Stir in the diced apple, ground cinnamon, and chia seeds. Cook for an additional 5 minutes.
4. Remove from heat and let the oats sit for a minute.
5. Serve the oatmeal in bowls, topped with chopped walnuts.
6. Drizzle with honey or maple syrup if desired.

Nutrition Info per Serving (Serves 4):

- Calories: 250
- Protein: 7g
- Carbohydrates: 40g
- Dietary Fiber: 6g
- Sugars: 10g
- Total Fat: 9g
- Saturated Fat: 1g
- Sodium: 10mg

Servings: 4 Cooking Time: 30 minutes

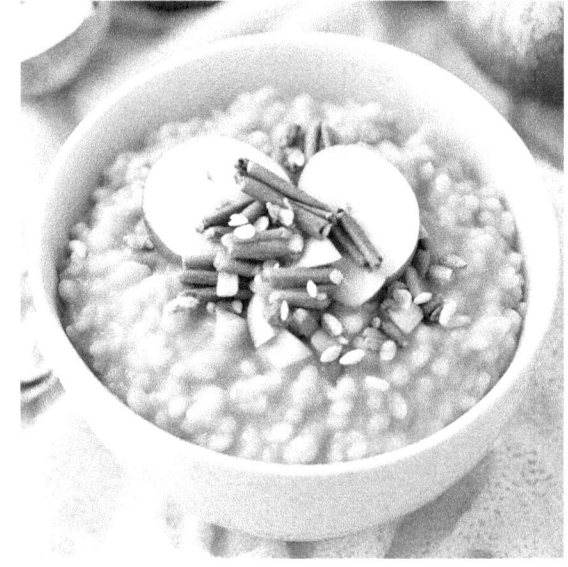

16. Muesli with Skim Milk

Ingredients:

- 1 cup rolled oats
- 1/4 cup chopped almonds
- 1/4 cup raisins
- 1/4 cup dried apricots, chopped
- 1/4 cup sunflower seeds
- 1 teaspoon ground cinnamon
- 2 cups skim milk

Instructions:

1. In a large bowl, combine the rolled oats, chopped almonds, raisins, chopped dried apricots, sunflower seeds, and ground cinnamon.
2. Divide the muesli mixture into four bowls.
3. Pour 1/2 cup of skim milk over each serving.
4. Serve immediately or refrigerate overnight for a softer texture.

Nutrition Info per Serving (Serves 4):

- Calories: 250
- Protcin: 9g
- Carbohydrates: 42g
- Dietary Fiber: 6g
- Sugars: 18g
- Total Fat: 7g
- Saturated Fat: 1g
- Sodium: 70mg

Servings: 4 Cooking Time: 5 minutes

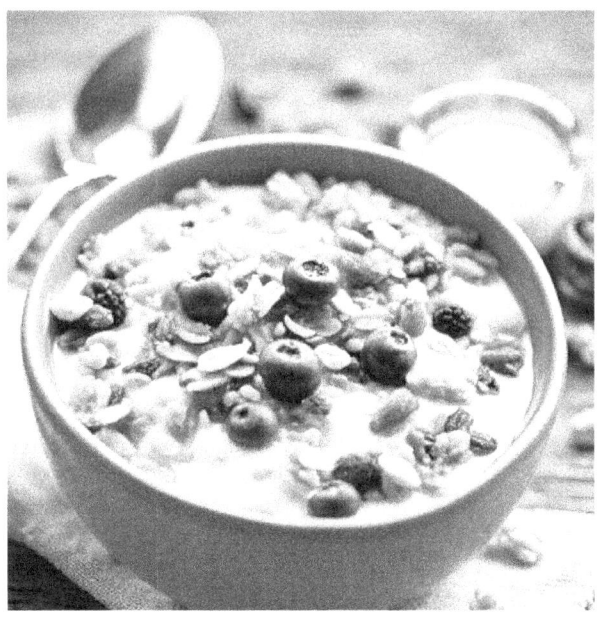

17. Mixed Berry Compote with Yogurt

Ingredients:

- 2 cups mixed fresh berries (strawberries, blueberries, raspberries)
- 1 tablespoon honey or maple syrup
- 1 teaspoon lemon juice
- 2 cups plain Greek yogurt
- 1/4 cup chopped walnuts

Instructions:

1. In a saucepan over medium heat, combine the mixed berries, honey or maple syrup, and lemon juice.
2. Cook, stirring occasionally, until the berries break down and the mixture thickens, about 10 minutes.
3. Remove from heat and let cool slightly.
4. Divide the Greek yogurt into four bowls.
5. Spoon the berry compote over the yogurt and sprinkle with chopped walnuts.
6. Serve immediately.

Nutrition Info per Serving (Serves 4):

- Calories: 200
- Protein: 10g
- Carbohydrates: 27g
- Dietary Fiber: 5g
- Sugars: 20g
- Total Fat: 7g
- Saturated Fat: 2g
- Sodium: 60mg

Servings: 4 Cooking Time: 15 minutes

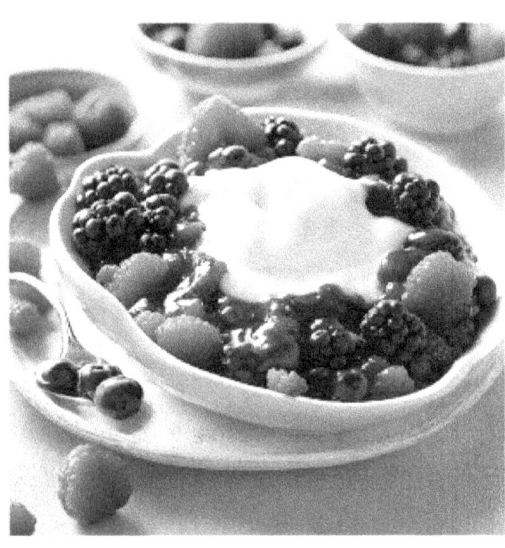

18. Pistachio and Peach Yogurt

Ingredients:

- 2 cups plain Greek yogurt
- 2 ripe peaches, pitted and sliced
- 1/4 cup shelled pistachios, chopped
- 1 tablespoon honey or maple syrup
- 1 teaspoon ground cinnamon

Instructions:

1. Divide the Greek yogurt into four bowls.
2. Top each bowl with peach slices.
3. Sprinkle with chopped pistachios and ground cinnamon.
4. Drizzle with honey or maple syrup.
5. Serve immediately.

Nutrition Info per Serving (Serves 4):

- Calories: 230
- Protein: 11g
- Carbohydrates: 26g
- Dietary Fiber: 3g
- Sugars: 20g
- Total Fat: 9g
- Saturated Fat: 2g
- Sodium: 50mg

Servings: 4 Cooking Time: 5 minutes

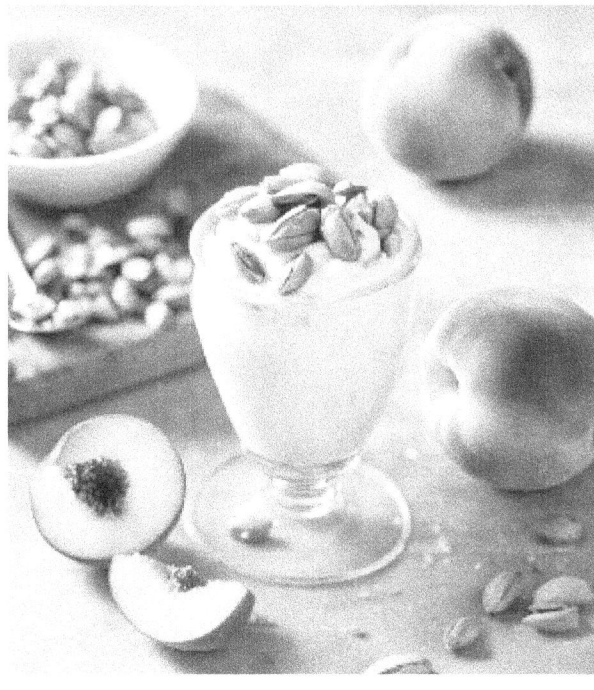

19. Spinach and Mushroom Toast

Ingredients:

- 4 slices whole grain bread
- 1 tablespoon olive oil
- 1 cup sliced mushrooms
- 1 cup fresh spinach, chopped
- 1/4 cup crumbled feta cheese
- 1/2 teaspoon garlic powder
- Freshly ground black pepper, to taste

Instructions:

1. Toast the whole grain bread slices until golden brown.
2. Heat olive oil in a skillet over medium heat.
3. Add the sliced mushrooms and cook for 3-4 minutes until tender.
4. Add the chopped spinach and cook until wilted, about 2 minutes.
5. Sprinkle with garlic powder and black pepper, and cook for another minute.
6. Spoon the spinach and mushroom mixture onto the toasted bread.
7. Sprinkle with crumbled feta cheese.
8. Serve immediately.

Nutrition Info per Serving (Serves 4):

- Calories: 180
- Protein: 7g
- Carbohydrates: 22g
- Dietary Fiber: 4g
- Sugars: 3g
- Total Fat: 8g
- Saturated Fat: 2g
- Sodium: 250mg

Servings: 4 Cooking Time: 10 minutes

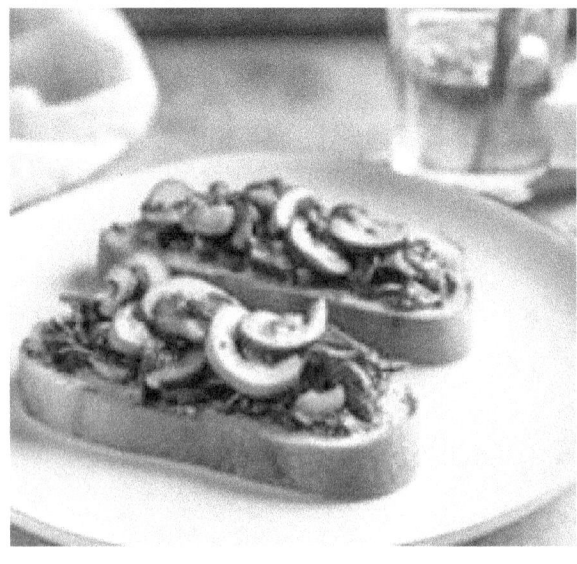

20. Buckwheat Porridge

Ingredients:
- 1 cup buckwheat groats
- 2 cups water
- 1 cup unsweetened almond milk
- 1 tablespoon chia seeds
- 1 teaspoon ground cinnamon
- 1 tablespoon honey or maple syrup
- 1/4 cup fresh blueberries
- 1/4 cup chopped walnuts

Instructions:
1. In a medium saucepan, bring the water to a boil.
2. Add the buckwheat groats, reduce the heat to low, and simmer for about 15 minutes, or until tender.
3. Stir in the almond milk, chia seeds, ground cinnamon, and honey or maple syrup.
4. Cook for an additional 5 minutes, stirring occasionally.
5. Remove from heat and let the porridge sit for a minute.
6. Serve the porridge in bowls, topped with fresh blueberries and chopped walnuts.

Nutrition Info per Serving (Serves 2):
- Calories: 320
- Protein: 8g
- Carbohydrates: 50g
- Dietary Fiber: 8g
- Sugars: 12g
- Total Fat: 10g
- Saturated Fat: 1g
- Sodium: 10mg

Servings: 2 Cooking Time: 20 minutes

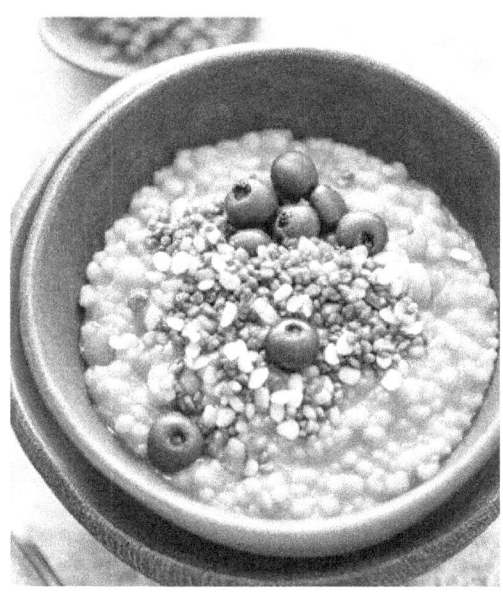

21. Egg and Avocado Salad

Ingredients:

- 4 large eggs
- 1 ripe avocado, diced
- 1/4 cup diced red onion
- 1/4 cup chopped fresh cilantro
- 1 tablespoon olive oil
- 1 tablespoon lemon juice
- Freshly ground black pepper, to taste

Instructions:

1. Place the eggs in a saucepan and cover with water. Bring to a boil, then reduce the heat and simmer for 10 minutes.
2. Remove the eggs from the water and let them cool. Peel and chop the eggs.
3. In a medium bowl, combine the chopped eggs, diced avocado, red onion, and cilantro.
4. Drizzle with olive oil and lemon juice. Mix gently to combine.
5. Serve immediately.

Nutrition Info per Serving (Serves 2):

- Calories: 280
- Protein: 12g
- Carbohydrates: 10g
- Dietary Fiber: 7g
- Sugars: 1g
- Total Fat: 23g
- Saturated Fat: 4g
- Sodium: 120mg

Servings: 2 Cooking Time: 15 minutes

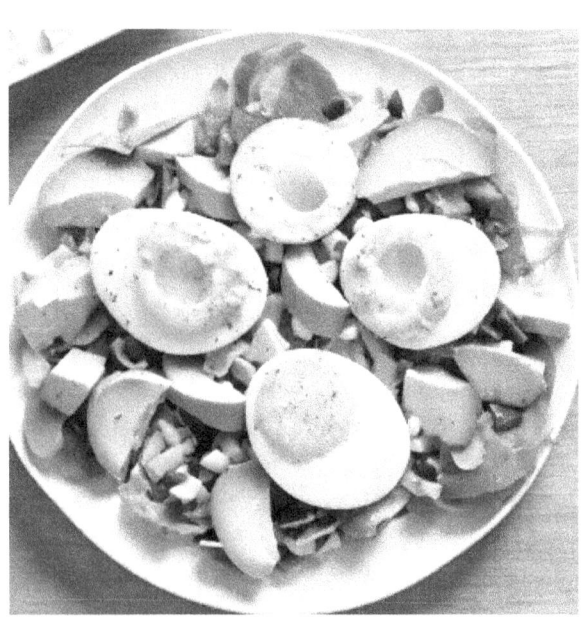

22. Peanut Butter Oatmeal

Ingredients:

- 1 cup rolled oats
- 2 cups water or unsweetened almond milk
- 2 tablespoons natural peanut butter
- 1 tablespoon chia seeds
- 1 teaspoon ground cinnamon
- 1 tablespoon honey or maple syrup (optional)
- 1/4 cup sliced bananas

Instructions:

1. In a medium saucepan, bring the water or almond milk to a boil.
2. Add the rolled oats and reduce the heat to medium-low. Cook, stirring occasionally, for about 5 minutes or until the oats are tender and the liquid is absorbed.
3. Stir in the peanut butter, chia seeds, and ground cinnamon until well combined.
4. Remove from heat and let the oatmeal sit for a minute.
5. Serve the oatmeal in bowls, topped with sliced bananas and drizzled with honey or maple syrup if desired.

Nutrition Info per Serving (Serves 2):

- Calories: 330
- Protein: 10g
- Carbohydrates: 45g
- Dietary Fiber: 8g
- Sugars: 12g
- Total Fat: 13g
- Saturated Fat: 2g
- Sodium: 60mg

Servings: 2 Cooking Time: 10 minutes

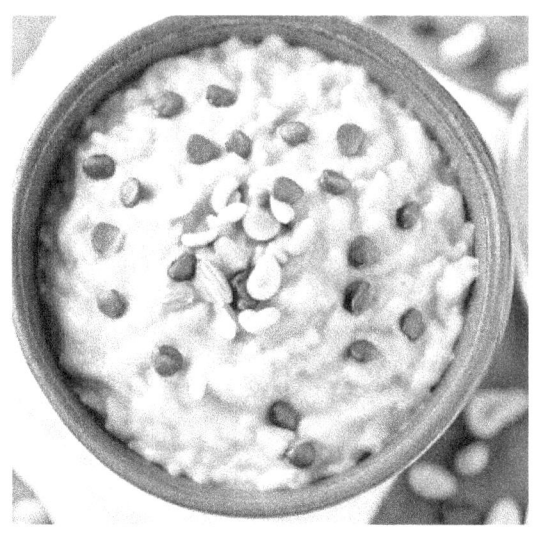

23. Veggie and Herb Cream Cheese Spread

Ingredients:

- 8 ounces low-fat cream cheese, softened
- 1/2 cup finely chopped red bell pepper
- 1/2 cup finely chopped cucumber
- 1/4 cup finely chopped green onions
- 2 tablespoons chopped fresh dill
- 1 tablespoon lemon juice
- Freshly ground black pepper, to taste

Instructions:

1. In a medium bowl, combine the softened cream cheese, chopped red bell pepper, cucumber, green onions, and fresh dill.
2. Add the lemon juice and black pepper.
3. Mix well until all ingredients are evenly distributed.
4. Serve immediately with whole grain crackers or as a spread on whole grain bread.

Nutrition Info per Serving (Serves 8):

- Calories: 70
- Protein: 3g
- Carbohydrates: 3g
- Dietary Fiber: 0.5g
- Sugars: 1g
- Total Fat: 5g
- Saturated Fat: 3g
- Sodium: 95mg

Servings: 8 Cooking Time: 10 minutes

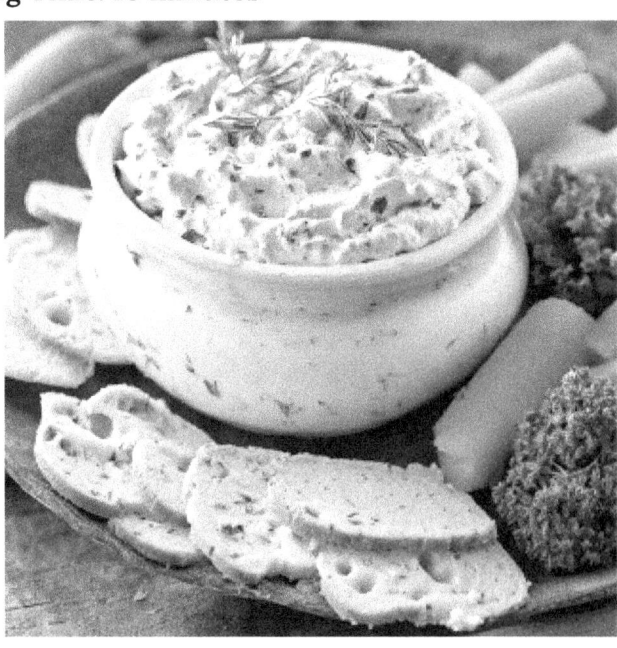

24. Beet and Berry Juice

Ingredients:
- 2 medium beets, peeled and chopped
- 1 cup mixed berries (strawberries, blueberries, raspberries)
- 1 apple, cored and chopped
- 1 tablespoon lemon juice
- 1 cup water

Instructions:
1. Place the beets, mixed berries, apple, lemon juice, and water in a blender.
2. Blend until smooth.
3. Strain the juice through a fine mesh sieve or cheesecloth to remove pulp, if desired.
4. Serve immediately.

Nutrition Info per Serving (Serves 2):
- Calories: 120
- Protein: 2g
- Carbohydrates: 29g
- Dietary Fiber: 5g
- Sugars: 20g
- Total Fat: 0.5g
- Saturated Fat: 0g
- Sodium: 50mg

Servings: 2 Cooking Time: 10 minutes

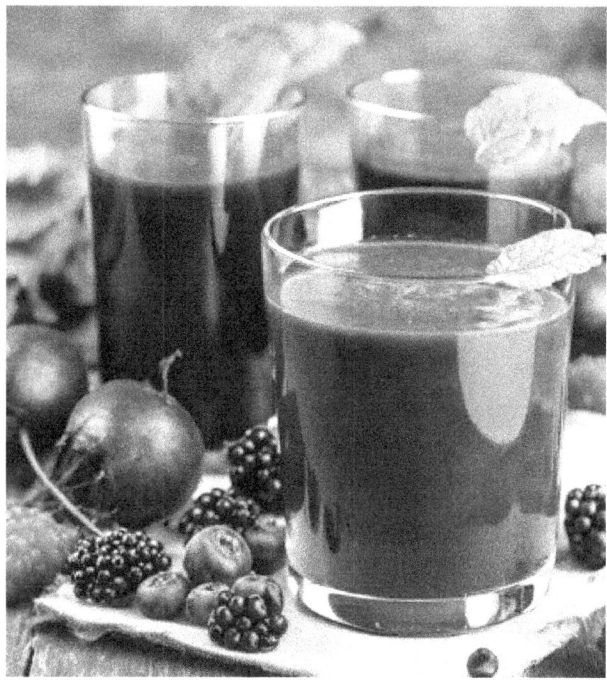

25. Spinach and Citrus Salad

Ingredients:

- 4 cups fresh spinach, washed and chopped
- 1 orange, peeled and segmented
- 1 grapefruit, peeled and segmented
- 1/4 cup sliced red onion
- 1/4 cup sliced almonds
- 1 tablespoon olive oil
- 1 tablespoon balsamic vinegar
- Freshly ground black pepper, to taste

Instructions:

1. In a large bowl, combine the chopped spinach, orange segments, grapefruit segments, and sliced red onion.
2. Drizzle with olive oil and balsamic vinegar.
3. Toss to combine.
4. Sprinkle with sliced almonds.
5. Serve immediately.

Nutrition Info per Serving (Serves 2):

- Calories: 180
- Protein: 3g
- Carbohydrates: 20g
- Dietary Fiber: 6g
- Sugars: 12g
- Total Fat: 10g
- Saturated Fat: 1g
- Sodium: 20mg

Servings: 2 Cooking Time: 10 minutes

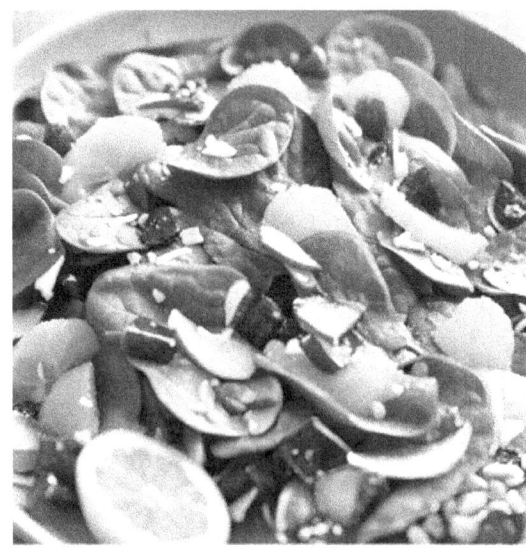

Poultry Recipes

1. Grilled Chicken with Avocado Salsa

Ingredients:

- 4 boneless, skinless chicken breasts
- 2 tablespoons olive oil
- 1 teaspoon garlic powder
- 1 teaspoon cumin
- 1 teaspoon paprika
- 1/2 teaspoon dried oregano
- 2 avocados, diced
- 1 cup cherry tomatoes, halved
- 1/4 cup red onion, finely chopped
- 1/4 cup fresh cilantro, chopped
- 1 tablespoon lime juice

Instructions:

1. In a small bowl, mix the olive oil, garlic powder, cumin, paprika, and oregano.
2. Rub the chicken breasts with the spice mixture and let them marinate for at least 15 minutes.
3. Preheat the grill to medium-high heat. Grill the chicken breasts for 6-8 minutes per side, or until fully cooked.
4. While the chicken is grilling, combine the diced avocados, cherry tomatoes, red onion, cilantro, and lime juice in a bowl. Mix gently.
5. Serve the grilled chicken topped with the avocado salsa.

Nutrition Info per Serving (Serves 4):

- Calories: 350
- Protein: 30g
- Carbohydrates: 12g
- Dietary Fiber: 6g
- Sugars: 2g
- Total Fat: 21g
- Saturated Fat: 3g
- Sodium: 100mg

Servings: 4 Cooking Time: 20 minutes

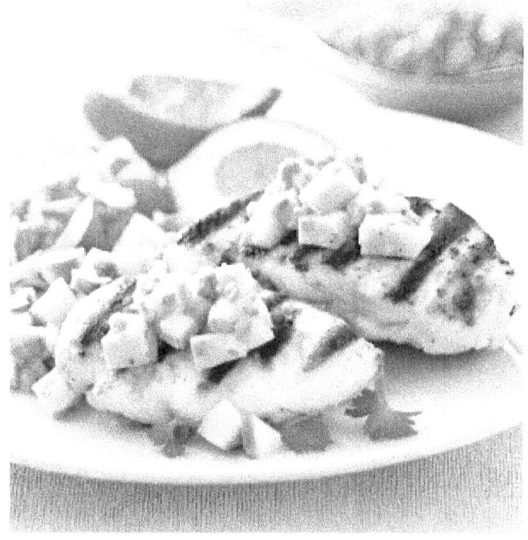

2. Turmeric Chicken Stir-Fry

Ingredients:

- 2 tablespoons olive oil
- 1 pound boneless, skinless chicken breast, thinly sliced
- 1 teaspoon ground turmeric
- 1 teaspoon garlic powder
- 1 teaspoon onion powder
- 1 red bell pepper, sliced
- 1 yellow bell pepper, sliced
- 1 cup broccoli florets
- 1/2 cup sliced carrots
- 2 tablespoons low-sodium soy sauce
- 1 tablespoon rice vinegar
- 1 teaspoon sesame seeds

Instructions:

1. In a large skillet, heat 1 tablespoon of olive oil over medium-high heat.
2. Add the sliced chicken, turmeric, garlic powder, and onion powder. Cook for 5-7 minutes until the chicken is browned and cooked through.
3. Remove the chicken from the skillet and set aside.
4. In the same skillet, add the remaining olive oil. Add the bell peppers, broccoli, and carrots. Stir-fry for 5-7 minutes until the vegetables are tender-crisp.
5. Return the chicken to the skillet. Add the soy sauce and rice vinegar, and stir to combine. Cook for another 2-3 minutes.
6. Sprinkle with sesame seeds and serve immediately.

Nutrition Info per Serving (Serves 4):

- Calories: 280
- Protein: 27g
- Carbohydrates: 12g
- Dietary Fiber: 4g
- Sugars: 5g
- Total Fat: 12g
- Saturated Fat: 2g
- Sodium: 400mg

Servings: 4 Cooking Time: 20 minutes

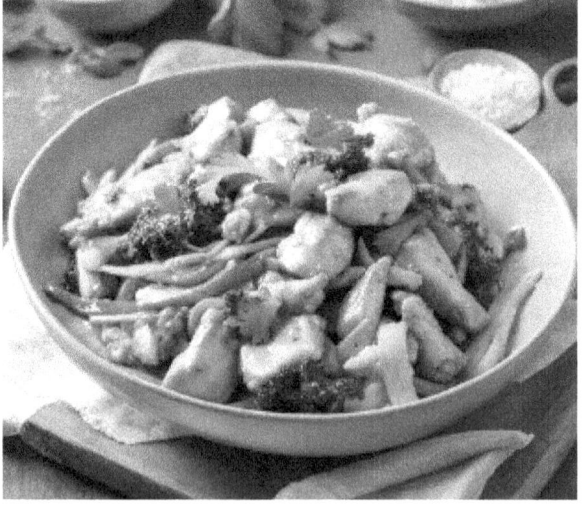

3. Lemon Herb Roasted Chicken

Ingredients:

- 1 whole chicken (about 4 pounds)
- 3 tablespoons olive oil
- 1 lemon, sliced
- 4 cloves garlic, minced
- 1 tablespoon dried rosemary
- 1 tablespoon dried thyme
- 1 tablespoon dried oregano
- 1 cup low-sodium chicken broth

Instructions:

1. Preheat the oven to 375°F (190°C).
2. In a small bowl, combine the olive oil, minced garlic, rosemary, thyme, and oregano.
3. Rub the herb mixture all over the chicken, including under the skin.
4. Place the lemon slices inside the cavity of the chicken.
5. Place the chicken in a roasting pan and pour the chicken broth into the pan.
6. Roast the chicken for about 1.5 hours, or until the internal temperature reaches 165°F (75°C) and the skin is golden brown.
7. Let the chicken rest for 10 minutes before carving and serving.

Nutrition Info per Serving (Serves 6):

- Calories: 350
- Protein: 30g
- Carbohydrates: 3g
- Dietary Fiber: 1g
- Sugars: 0g
- Total Fat: 23g
- Saturated Fat: 6g
- Sodium: 150mg

Servings: 6 Cooking Time: 1.5 hours

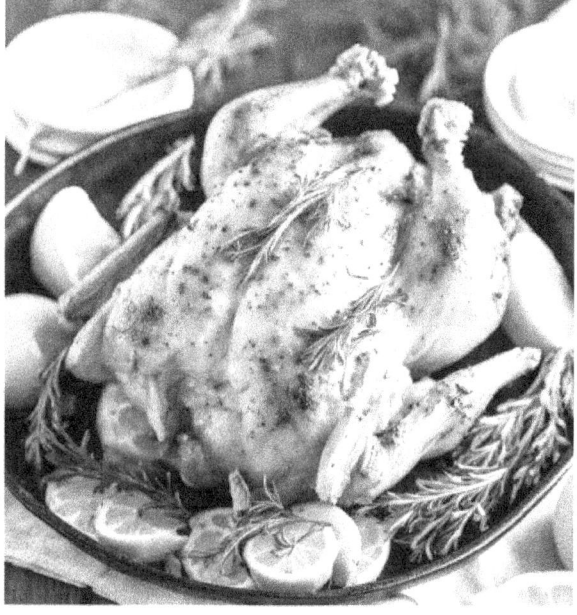

4. Chicken and Spinach Soup

Ingredients:

- 1 tablespoon olive oil
- 1 pound boneless, skinless chicken breast, diced
- 1 onion, chopped
- 2 cloves garlic, minced
- 2 carrots, sliced
- 2 celery stalks, sliced
- 6 cups low-sodium chicken broth
- 2 cups fresh spinach, chopped
- 1 teaspoon dried thyme
- 1 teaspoon dried basil
- 1/4 teaspoon black pepper

Instructions:

1. In a large pot, heat the olive oil over medium heat.
2. Add the diced chicken and cook until browned, about 5-7 minutes. Remove the chicken and set aside.
3. In the same pot, add the chopped onion and garlic. Cook for 3-4 minutes until softened.
4. Add the sliced carrots and celery, and cook for another 5 minutes.
5. Pour in the chicken broth and add the cooked chicken back to the pot.
6. Stir in the dried thyme, basil, and black pepper. Bring to a boil, then reduce the heat and simmer for 15 minutes.
7. Add the chopped spinach and cook for an additional 5 minutes until wilted.
8. Serve hot.

Nutrition Info per Serving (Serves 4):

- Calories: 210
- Protein: 25g
- Carbohydrates: 10g
- Dietary Fiber: 2g
- Sugars: 4g
- Total Fat: 8g
- Saturated Fat: 1.5g
- Sodium: 250mg

Servings: 4 Cooking Time: 30 minutes

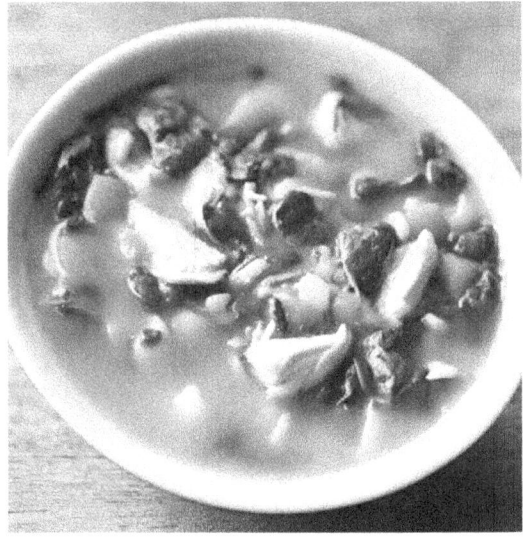

5. Balsamic Chicken Salad

Ingredients:

- 4 boneless, skinless chicken breasts
- 2 tablespoons olive oil
- 1/4 cup balsamic vinegar
- 1 teaspoon garlic powder
- 1 teaspoon dried oregano
- 4 cups mixed salad greens
- 1 cup cherry tomatoes, halved
- 1/4 cup red onion, thinly sliced
- 1/4 cup crumbled feta cheese
- 1/4 cup walnuts, chopped

Instructions:

1. In a small bowl, mix the olive oil, balsamic vinegar, garlic powder, and oregano.
2. Marinate the chicken breasts in the mixture for at least 15 minutes.
3. Preheat a grill or skillet over medium-high heat. Grill the chicken breasts for 6-8 minutes per side, or until fully cooked. Let the chicken rest for 5 minutes, then slice.
4. In a large bowl, combine the mixed salad greens, cherry tomatoes, red onion, feta cheese, and walnuts.
5. Top the salad with the sliced chicken and drizzle with additional balsamic vinegar if desired.
6. Serve immediately.

Nutrition Info per Serving (Serves 4):

- Calories: 350
- Protein: 30g
- Carbohydrates: 12g
- Dietary Fiber: 4g
- Sugars: 5g
- Total Fat: 20g
- Saturated Fat: 4g
- Sodium: 220mg

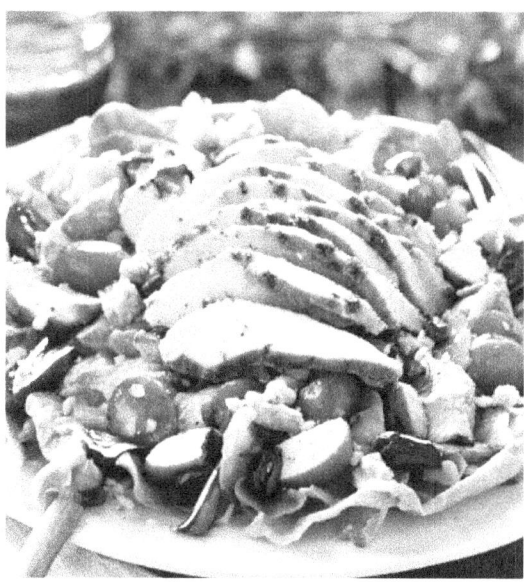

Servings: 4 Cooking Time: 25 minutes

6. Chicken Cauliflower Fried Rice

Ingredients:

- 1 pound boneless, skinless chicken breast, diced
- 2 tablespoons olive oil
- 1 small onion, chopped
- 2 cloves garlic, minced
- 1 head cauliflower, riced
- 1 cup frozen peas and carrots
- 2 large eggs, beaten
- 3 tablespoons low-sodium soy sauce
- 1 teaspoon ground ginger
- 1/4 cup green onions, chopped

Instructions:

1. Heat 1 tablespoon of olive oil in a large skillet over medium-high heat. Add the diced chicken and cook for 5-7 minutes until browned and cooked through. Remove the chicken and set aside.
2. In the same skillet, add the remaining olive oil and sauté the chopped onion and garlic until fragrant, about 2-3 minutes.
3. Add the riced cauliflower and cook for 5 minutes, stirring frequently.
4. Stir in the peas and carrots, and cook for another 2 minutes.
5. Push the vegetables to one side of the skillet and pour the beaten eggs into the other side. Scramble the eggs until fully cooked, then mix them into the vegetables.
6. Return the chicken to the skillet, and add the soy sauce and ground ginger. Stir well to combine.
7. Sprinkle with chopped green onions and serve immediately.

Nutrition Info per Serving (Serves 4):

- Calories: 300
- Protein: 27g
- Carbohydrates: 14g
- Dietary Fiber: 5g
- Sugars: 5g
- Total Fat: 14g
- Saturated Fat: 3g
- Sodium: 450mg

Servings: 4 Cooking Time: 20 minutes

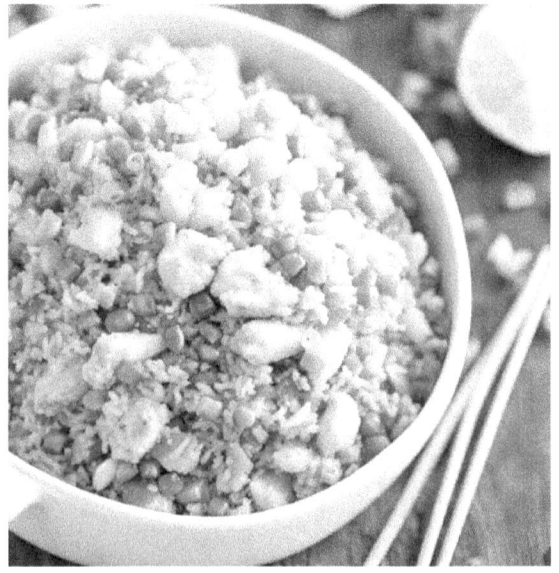

7. Greek Chicken Skewers

Ingredients:

- 1 pound boneless, skinless chicken breast, cut into cubes
- 2 tablespoons olive oil
- 2 tablespoons lemon juice
- 1 teaspoon dried oregano
- 1 teaspoon garlic powder
- 1 red bell pepper, cut into squares
- 1 green bell pepper, cut into squares
- 1 red onion, cut into squares

Instructions:

1. In a bowl, combine olive oil, lemon juice, oregano, and garlic powder. Add chicken cubes and marinate for at least 30 minutes.
2. Preheat the grill to medium-high heat.
3. Thread the chicken, red bell pepper, green bell pepper, and red onion onto skewers.
4. Grill the skewers for about 10-12 minutes, turning occasionally, until the chicken is fully cooked and vegetables are tender.
5. Serve immediately.

Nutrition Info per Serving (Serves 4):

- Calories: 220
- Protein: 25g
- Carbohydrates: 8g
- Dietary Fiber: 2g
- Sugars: 4g
- Total Fat: 10g
- Saturated Fat: 2g
- Sodium: 120mg

Servings: 4 Cooking Time: 20 minutes (plus marinating time)

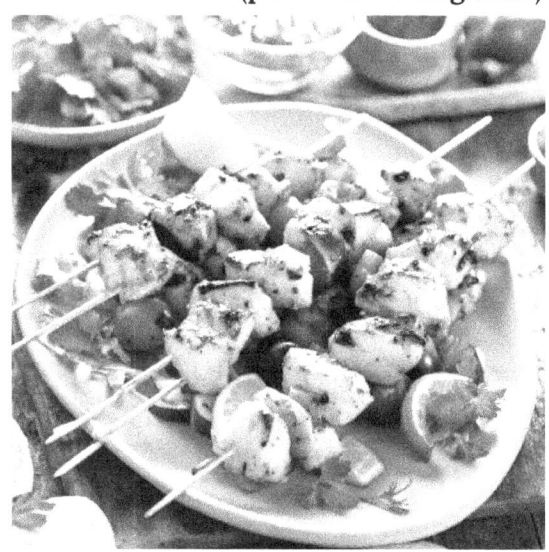

8. Mediterranean Chicken Wrap

Ingredients:

- 4 whole grain tortillas
- 1 pound boneless, skinless chicken breast, cooked and sliced
- 1 cup hummus
- 1 cup mixed greens
- 1/2 cup cherry tomatoes, halved
- 1/4 cup red onion, thinly sliced
- 1/4 cup crumbled feta cheese
- 2 tablespoons olive oil
- 1 tablespoon lemon juice
- 1 teaspoon dried oregano

Instructions:

1. In a small bowl, mix olive oil, lemon juice, and oregano.
2. Toss the sliced chicken with the dressing.
3. Lay out the tortillas and spread 1/4 cup hummus on each.
4. Divide the mixed greens, cherry tomatoes, red onion, feta cheese, and seasoned chicken among the tortillas.
5. Roll up the tortillas and serve immediately.

Nutrition Info per Serving (Serves 4):

- Calories: 380
- Protein: 30g
- Carbohydrates: 32g
- Dietary Fiber: 6g
- Sugars: 4g
- Total Fat: 15g
- Saturated Fat: 3g
- Sodium: 450mg

Servings: 4 Cooking Time: 10 minutes

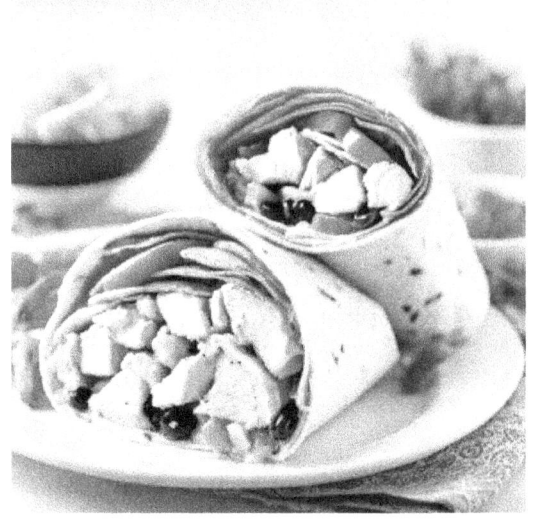

9. Sesame Chicken and Broccoli

Ingredients:

- 1 pound boneless, skinless chicken breast, cut into strips
- 3 tablespoons olive oil, divided
- 1 tablespoon sesame oil
- 3 tablespoons low-sodium soy sauce
- 1 tablespoon honey
- 1 teaspoon ground ginger
- 4 cups broccoli florets
- 1 tablespoon sesame seeds

Instructions:

1. Heat 2 tablespoons of olive oil in a large skillet over medium-high heat. Add the chicken strips and cook for 5-7 minutes until browned and cooked through. Remove the chicken and set aside.
2. In the same skillet, add the remaining olive oil and sesame oil. Add the broccoli florets and cook for 4-5 minutes until tender-crisp.
3. In a small bowl, mix the soy sauce, honey, and ground ginger. Add the cooked chicken back to the skillet and pour the sauce over it. Stir well to combine.
4. Cook for another 2-3 minutes until the sauce thickens slightly.
5. Sprinkle with sesame seeds and serve immediately.

Nutrition Info per Serving (Serves 4):

- Calories: 280
- Protein: 26g
- Carbohydrates: 12g
- Dietary Fiber: 4g
- Sugars: 6g
- Total Fat: 14g
- Saturated Fat: 2g
- Sodium: 500mg

Servings: 4 Cooking Time: 15 minutes

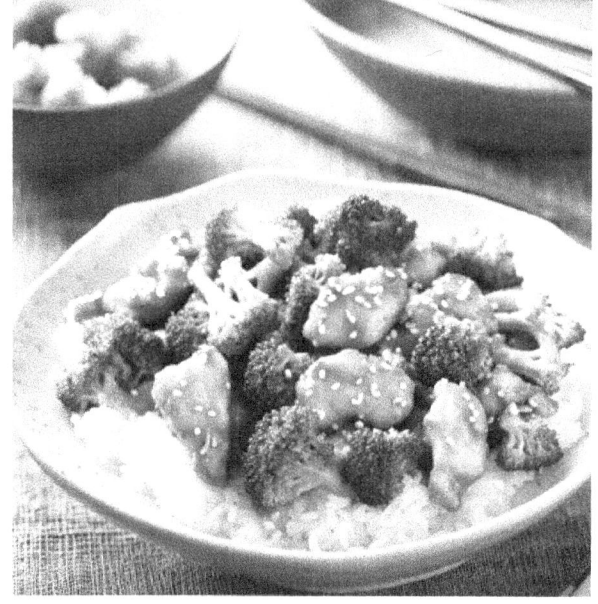

10. Chicken and Barley Soup

Ingredients:

- 1 tablespoon olive oil
- 1 pound boneless, skinless chicken breast, diced
- 1 onion, chopped
- 2 cloves garlic, minced
- 2 carrots, sliced
- 2 celery stalks, sliced
- 6 cups low-sodium chicken broth
- 1 cup pearl barley
- 1 teaspoon dried thyme
- 1 teaspoon dried basil
- 2 cups fresh spinach, chopped
- 1/4 teaspoon black pepper

Instructions:

1. In a large pot, heat the olive oil over medium heat. Add the diced chicken and cook for 5-7 minutes until browned and cooked through. Remove the chicken and set aside.
2. In the same pot, add the chopped onion and garlic. Cook for 3-4 minutes until softened.
3. Add the sliced carrots and celery, and cook for another 5 minutes.
4. Pour in the chicken broth and add the pearl barley, dried thyme, and dried basil. Bring to a boil.
5. Reduce the heat and simmer for 30-40 minutes, or until the barley is tender.
6. Add the cooked chicken back to the pot, along with the chopped spinach and black pepper. Cook for another 5 minutes until the spinach is wilted.
7. Serve hot.

Nutrition Info per Serving (Serves 6):

- Calories: 250
- Protein: 25g
- Carbohydrates: 30g
- Dietary Fiber: 6g
- Sugars: 4g
- Total Fat: 6g
- Saturated Fat: 1g
- Sodium: 200mg

Servings: 6 Cooking Time: 1 hour

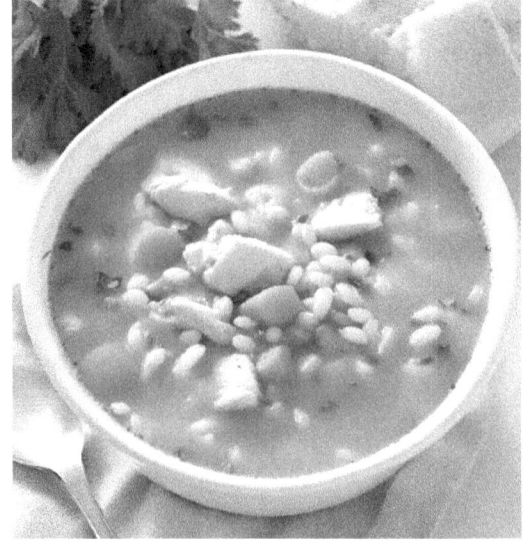

11. Chicken Piccata with Capers

Ingredients:

- 4 boneless, skinless chicken breasts
- 1/4 cup whole wheat flour
- 2 tablespoons olive oil
- 1/4 cup fresh lemon juice
- 1/2 cup low-sodium chicken broth
- 2 tablespoons capers, rinsed and drained
- 1 tablespoon chopped fresh parsley

Instructions:

1. Pound the chicken breasts to an even thickness and dredge them lightly in the flour.
2. Heat the olive oil in a large skillet over medium-high heat.
3. Add the chicken breasts and cook for 5-6 minutes per side, until golden brown and cooked through. Remove the chicken from the skillet and set aside.
4. In the same skillet, add the lemon juice, chicken broth, and capers. Bring to a boil, scraping up any browned bits from the bottom of the pan.
5. Return the chicken to the skillet and simmer for 5 minutes, spooning the sauce over the chicken.
6. Sprinkle with chopped parsley and serve immediately.

Nutrition Info per Serving (Serves 4):

- Calories: 280
- Protein: 28g
- Carbohydrates: 8g
- Dietary Fiber: 1g
- Sugars: 0g
- Total Fat: 14g
- Saturated Fat: 2g
- Sodium: 220mg

Servings: 4 Cooking Time: 25 minutes

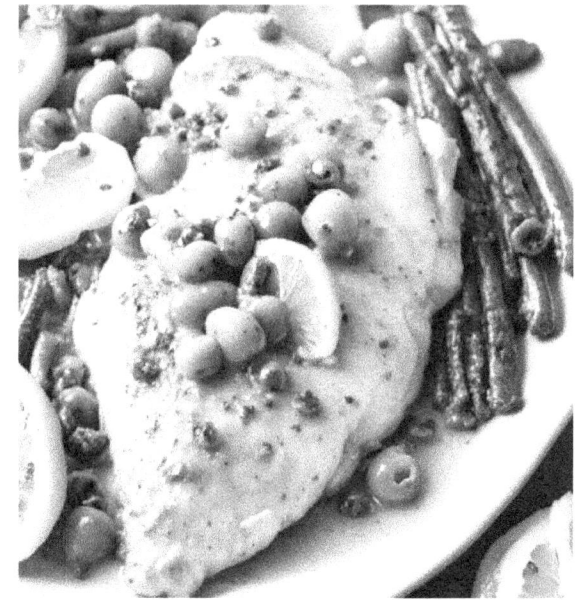

12. Moroccan Chicken Stew

Ingredients:

- 2 tablespoons olive oil
- 1 pound boneless, skinless chicken thighs, cut into chunks
- 1 onion, chopped
- 2 cloves garlic, minced
- 2 carrots, sliced
- 2 celery stalks, sliced
- 1 teaspoon ground cumin
- 1 teaspoon ground cinnamon
- 1 teaspoon ground ginger
- 1/2 teaspoon turmeric
- 1/2 teaspoon paprika
- 1 can (14.5 oz) diced tomatoes, no salt added
- 4 cups low-sodium chicken broth
- 1 cup chickpeas, drained and rinsed
- 1/2 cup dried apricots, chopped
- 1/4 cup chopped fresh cilantro

Instructions:

1. Heat 1 tablespoon of olive oil in a large pot over medium-high heat. Add the chicken and cook until browned, about 5-7 minutes. Remove the chicken and set aside.
2. In the same pot, add the remaining olive oil and sauté the onion and garlic until softened, about 3-4 minutes.
3. Add the carrots, celery, cumin, cinnamon, ginger, turmeric, and paprika. Cook for 2-3 minutes until fragrant.
4. Stir in the diced tomatoes, chicken broth, chickpeas, and dried apricots.
5. Return the chicken to the pot and bring to a boil. Reduce the heat and simmer for 30 minutes.
6. Garnish with chopped fresh cilantro and serve.

Nutrition Info per Serving (Serves 4):

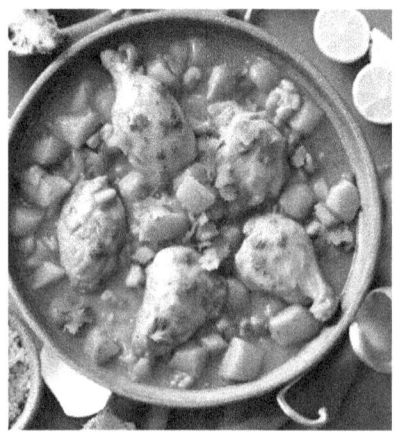

- Calories: 350
- Protein: 28g
- Carbohydrates: 30g
- Dietary Fiber: 8g
- Sugars: 12g
- Total Fat: 12g
- Saturated Fat: 2g
- Sodium: 320mg

Servings: 4 Cooking Time: 45 minutes

13. Tandoori Chicken

Ingredients:

- 1 pound boneless, skinless chicken thighs
- 1 cup plain Greek yogurt
- 2 tablespoons lemon juice
- 2 cloves garlic, minced
- 1 tablespoon grated ginger
- 1 teaspoon ground cumin
- 1 teaspoon ground coriander
- 1 teaspoon ground turmeric
- 1 teaspoon paprika
- 1/2 teaspoon ground black pepper
- 1/2 teaspoon ground cinnamon

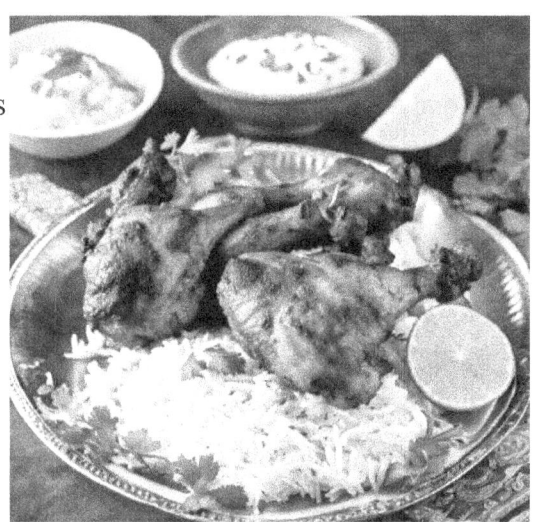

Instructions:

1. In a large bowl, combine the Greek yogurt, lemon juice, garlic, ginger, cumin, coriander, turmeric, paprika, black pepper, and cinnamon.
2. Add the chicken thighs to the marinade, making sure they are well coated. Marinate in the refrigerator for at least 2 hours or overnight.
3. Preheat the oven to 375°F (190°C). Place the marinated chicken thighs on a baking sheet lined with parchment paper.
4. Bake for 25-30 minutes, until the chicken is cooked through and slightly charred.
5. Serve immediately.

Nutrition Info per Serving (Serves 4):

- Calories: 230
- Protein: 25g
- Carbohydrates: 8g
- Dietary Fiber: 1g
- Sugars: 3g
- Total Fat: 10g
- Saturated Fat: 2g
- Sodium: 180mg

Servings: 4 Cooking Time: 30 minutes (plus marinating time)

14. Turkey Chili

Ingredients:

- 1 tablespoon olive oil
- 1 pound ground turkey
- 1 onion, chopped
- 2 cloves garlic, minced
- 1 red bell pepper, chopped
- 1 green bell pepper, chopped
- 1 can (14.5 oz) diced tomatoes, no salt added
- 1 can (15 oz) kidney beans, drained and rinsed
- 1 can (15 oz) black beans, drained and rinsed
- 2 cups low-sodium chicken broth
- 2 tablespoons chili powder
- 1 teaspoon ground cumin
- 1 teaspoon smoked paprika
- 1/4 teaspoon ground black pepper

Instructions:

1. Heat the olive oil in a large pot over medium-high heat. Add the ground turkey and cook until browned, about 5-7 minutes.
2. Add the chopped onion, garlic, red bell pepper, and green bell pepper. Cook for 5-7 minutes until vegetables are tender.
3. Stir in the diced tomatoes, kidney beans, black beans, chicken broth, chili powder, cumin, smoked paprika, and black pepper.
4. Bring to a boil, then reduce the heat and simmer for 30 minutes.
5. Serve hot.

Nutrition Info per Serving (Serves 6):

- Calories: 280
- Protein: 24g
- Carbohydrates: 30g
- Dietary Fiber: 10g
- Sugars: 6g
- Total Fat: 8g
- Saturated Fat: 2g
- Sodium: 320mg

Servings: 6 Cooking Time: 45 minutes

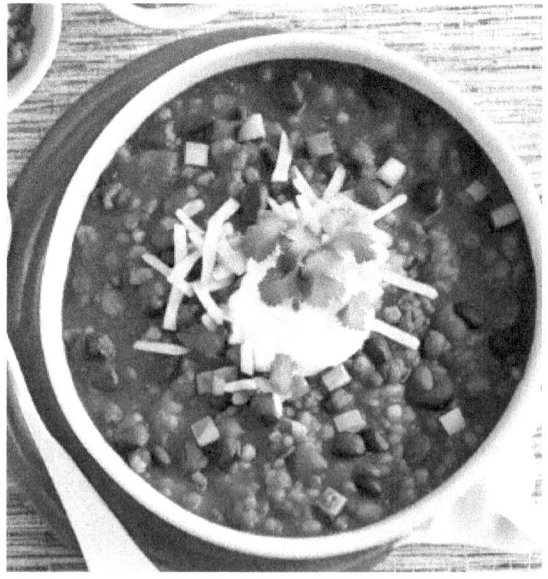

15. Turkey Meatballs in Tomato Basil Sauce

Ingredients:

- 1 pound ground turkey
- 1/4 cup whole wheat breadcrumbs
- 1/4 cup grated Parmesan cheese
- 1 large egg
- 2 cloves garlic, minced
- 1 tablespoon chopped fresh parsley
- 1 tablespoon olive oil
- 1 can (28 oz) crushed tomatoes, no salt added
- 1 teaspoon dried basil
- 1/2 teaspoon dried oregano
- 1/4 teaspoon ground black pepper
- 1/4 cup chopped fresh basil

Instructions:

1. In a large bowl, combine the ground turkey, breadcrumbs, Parmesan cheese, egg, minced garlic, and chopped parsley. Mix well and form into 1-inch meatballs.
2. Heat the olive oil in a large skillet over medium-high heat. Add the meatballs and cook for 5-7 minutes, turning occasionally, until browned on all sides.
3. In a large pot, combine the crushed tomatoes, dried basil, oregano, and black pepper. Bring to a simmer.
4. Add the browned meatballs to the tomato sauce and simmer for 20-25 minutes until the meatballs are cooked through.
5. Stir in the chopped fresh basil and serve immediately.

Nutrition Info per Serving (Serves 4):

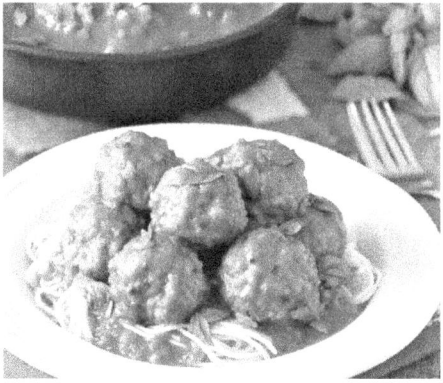

- Calories: 300
- Protein: 28g
- Carbohydrates: 14g
- Dietary Fiber: 4g
- Sugars: 6g
- Total Fat: 14g
- Saturated Fat: 4g
- Sodium: 320mg

Servings: 4 Cooking Time: 35 minutes

16. Turkey and Spinach Meatloaf

Ingredients:

- 1 pound ground turkey
- 1 cup fresh spinach, chopped
- 1/2 cup whole wheat breadcrumbs
- 1/4 cup grated Parmesan cheese
- 1 large egg
- 1 small onion, finely chopped
- 2 cloves garlic, minced
- 1 teaspoon dried oregano
- 1/2 teaspoon ground black pepper
- 1/2 cup low-sodium tomato sauce

Instructions:

1. Preheat the oven to 375°F (190°C).
2. In a large bowl, combine the ground turkey, chopped spinach, breadcrumbs, Parmesan cheese, egg, chopped onion, minced garlic, oregano, and black pepper. Mix well.
3. Transfer the mixture to a loaf pan and shape it into a loaf.
4. Spread the tomato sauce evenly over the top of the meatloaf.
5. Bake for 45-50 minutes, or until the meatloaf is cooked through and reaches an internal temperature of 165°F (75°C).
6. Let the meatloaf rest for 10 minutes before slicing and serving.

Nutrition Info per Serving (Serves 4):

- Calories: 250
- Protein: 28g
- Carbohydrates: 14g
- Dietary Fiber: 2g
- Sugars: 4g
- Total Fat: 10g
- Saturated Fat: 2g
- Sodium: 300mg

Servings: 4 Cooking Time: 60 minutes

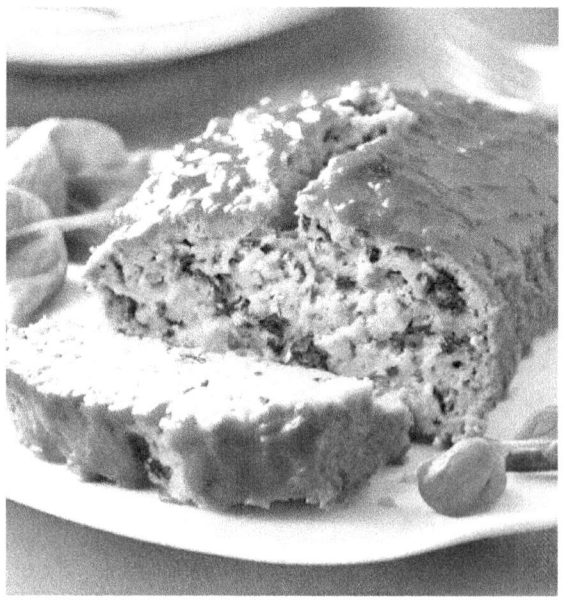

17. Smoked Turkey Salad

Ingredients:

- 2 cups mixed salad greens
- 1 cup smoked turkey breast, chopped
- 1/2 cup cherry tomatoes, halved
- 1/4 cup red onion, thinly sliced
- 1/4 cup crumbled feta cheese
- 1/4 cup walnuts, chopped
- 2 tablespoons olive oil
- 1 tablespoon balsamic vinegar
- 1 teaspoon Dijon mustard
- 1/4 teaspoon ground black pepper

Instructions:

1. In a large bowl, combine the mixed salad greens, smoked turkey, cherry tomatoes, red onion, feta cheese, and walnuts.
2. In a small bowl, whisk together the olive oil, balsamic vinegar, Dijon mustard, and black pepper.
3. Drizzle the dressing over the salad and toss to combine.
4. Serve immediately.

Nutrition Info per Serving (Serves 2):

- Calories: 320
- Protein: 25g
- Carbohydrates: 10g
- Dietary Fiber: 3g
- Sugars: 4g
- Total Fat: 20g
- Saturated Fat: 4g
- Sodium: 450mg

Servings: 2 Cooking Time: 10 minutes

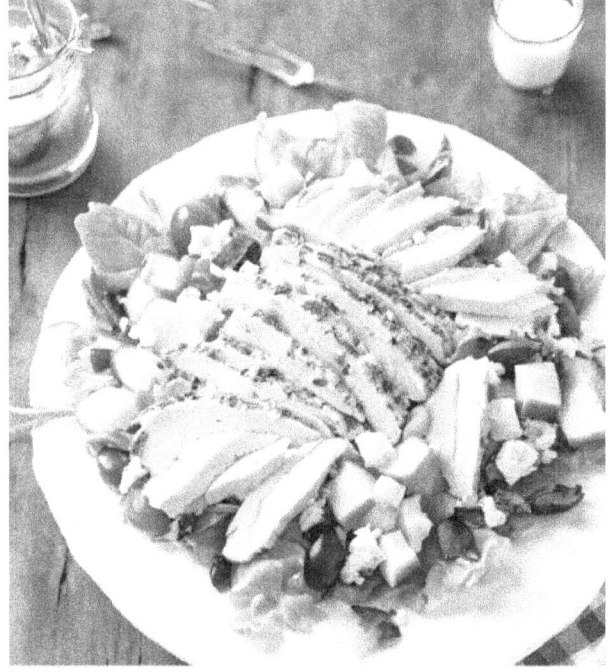

18. Turkey Sweet Potato Skillet

Ingredients:

- 1 pound ground turkey
- 2 tablespoons olive oil
- 1 large sweet potato, peeled and diced
- 1 small onion, chopped
- 2 cloves garlic, minced
- 1 red bell pepper, chopped
- 1 teaspoon ground cumin
- 1 teaspoon paprika
- 1/4 teaspoon ground black pepper
- 2 cups fresh spinach, chopped

Instructions:

1. Heat 1 tablespoon of olive oil in a large skillet over medium-high heat. Add the ground turkey and cook until browned, about 5-7 minutes. Remove the turkey and set aside.
2. In the same skillet, add the remaining olive oil and sauté the diced sweet potato for 5-7 minutes, until tender.
3. Add the chopped onion, minced garlic, and red bell pepper. Cook for another 5 minutes until the vegetables are softened.
4. Stir in the cooked turkey, ground cumin, paprika, and black pepper. Cook for 2-3 minutes until heated through.
5. Add the chopped spinach and cook for an additional 2 minutes, until wilted.
6. Serve immediately.

Nutrition Info per Serving (Serves 4):

- Calories: 350
- Protein: 28g
- Carbohydrates: 28g
- Dietary Fiber: 6g
- Sugars: 8g
- Total Fat: 15g
- Saturated Fat: 3g
- Sodium: 200mg

Servings: 4 Cooking Time: 25 minutes

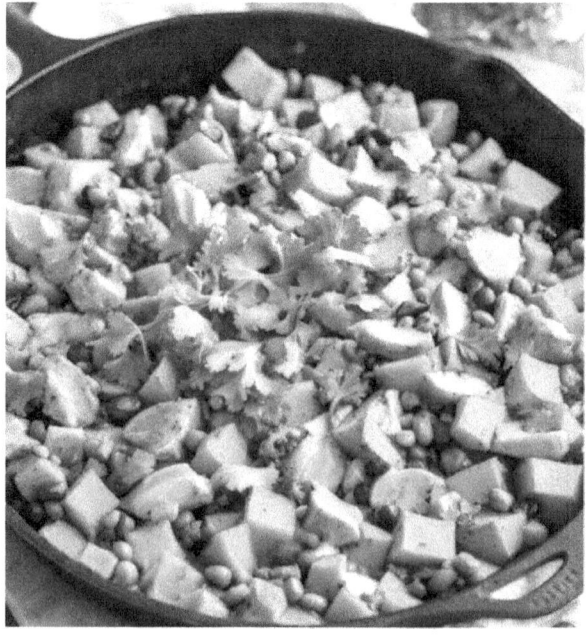

19. Baked Turkey and Eggplant Parmesan
Ingredients:
- 1 pound ground turkey
- 1 large eggplant, sliced into 1/4-inch rounds
- 2 tablespoons olive oil
- 1 onion, chopped
- 2 cloves garlic, minced
- 1 can (28 oz) crushed tomatoes, no salt added
- 1 teaspoon dried basil
- 1 teaspoon dried oregano
- 1/4 teaspoon ground black pepper
- 1/2 cup grated Parmesan cheese
- 1/2 cup shredded mozzarella cheese, part-skim

Instructions:
1. Preheat the oven to 375°F (190°C).
2. Sprinkle the eggplant slices with a little salt and let them sit for 10 minutes to draw out moisture. Pat them dry with a paper towel.
3. In a large skillet, heat 1 tablespoon of olive oil over medium heat. Add the chopped onion and garlic, and sauté until fragrant, about 3 minutes.
4. Add the ground turkey and cook until browned, about 5-7 minutes.
5. Stir in the crushed tomatoes, basil, oregano, and black pepper. Simmer for 10 minutes.
6. In another skillet, heat the remaining olive oil over medium-high heat. Add the eggplant slices and cook until lightly browned on both sides, about 3-4 minutes per side.
7. In a baking dish, layer half of the eggplant slices, then spread half of the turkey mixture over the eggplant. Sprinkle with half of the Parmesan cheese. Repeat with the remaining eggplant, turkey mixture, and Parmesan cheese.
8. Top with shredded mozzarella cheese.
9. Bake for 25-30 minutes, until the cheese is melted and bubbly.
10. Let rest for 5 minutes before serving.

Nutrition Info per Serving (Serves 4):
- Calories: 350
- Protein: 30g
- Carbohydrates: 20g
- Dietary Fiber: 7g
- Sugars: 10g
- Total Fat: 18g
- Saturated Fat: 6g
- Sodium: 380mg

Servings: 4 Cooking Time: 50 minutes

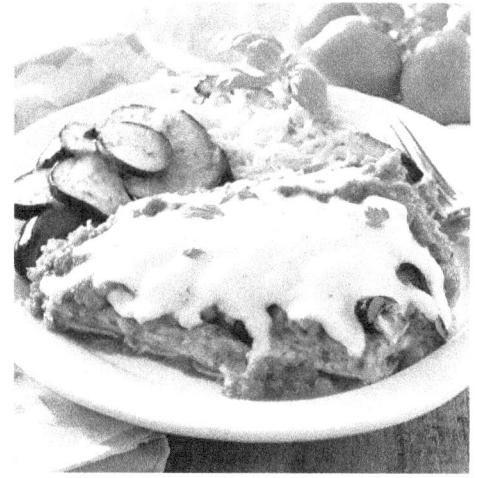

20. Italian Turkey and Zucchini Skillet

Ingredients:
- 1 pound ground turkey
- 2 tablespoons olive oil
- 1 onion, chopped
- 2 cloves garlic, minced
- 2 medium zucchinis, sliced into rounds
- 1 can (14.5 oz) diced tomatoes, no salt added
- 1 teaspoon dried basil
- 1 teaspoon dried oregano
- 1/4 teaspoon ground black pepper
- 1/4 cup grated Parmesan cheese

Instructions:
1. Heat 1 tablespoon of olive oil in a large skillet over medium-high heat. Add the ground turkey and cook until browned, about 5-7 minutes. Remove the turkey and set aside.
2. In the same skillet, add the remaining olive oil and sauté the chopped onion and minced garlic until softened, about 3-4 minutes.
3. Add the sliced zucchini and cook for 5 minutes until tender.
4. Stir in the diced tomatoes, basil, oregano, and black pepper. Cook for an additional 5 minutes.
5. Return the cooked turkey to the skillet and mix well. Cook for 2-3 minutes until heated through.
6. Sprinkle with grated Parmesan cheese and serve immediately.

Nutrition Info per Serving (Serves 4):
- Calories: 280
- Protein: 27g
- Carbohydrates: 12g
- Dietary Fiber: 4g
- Sugars: 6g
- Total Fat: 14g
- Saturated Fat: 3g
- Sodium: 280mg

Servings: 4 Cooking Time: 25 minutes

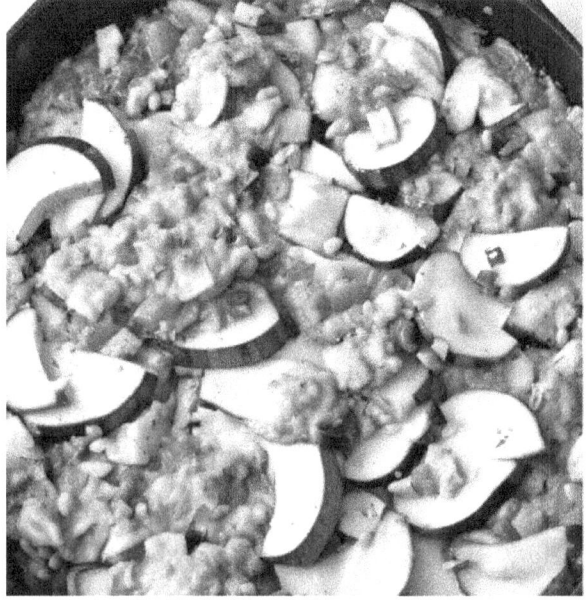

21. Turkey Taco Salad

Ingredients:

- 1 pound ground turkey
- 1 tablespoon olive oil
- 1 onion, chopped
- 2 cloves garlic, minced
- 1 tablespoon chili powder
- 1 teaspoon ground cumin
- 1 teaspoon paprika
- 1/4 teaspoon ground black pepper
- 4 cups mixed salad greens
- 1 cup cherry tomatoes, halved
- 1/2 cup red bell pepper, chopped
- 1/2 cup corn kernels (fresh or frozen, thawed)
- 1/4 cup black beans, rinsed and drained
- 1/4 cup shredded cheddar cheese, reduced-fat
- 1 avocado, sliced
- 1/4 cup salsa

Instructions:

1. In a large skillet, heat olive oil over medium-high heat. Add the ground turkey, chopped onion, and minced garlic. Cook until the turkey is browned and the onion is softened, about 5-7 minutes.
2. Stir in the chili powder, cumin, paprika, and black pepper. Cook for an additional 2-3 minutes until the spices are well blended.
3. In a large bowl, combine the mixed salad greens, cherry tomatoes, red bell pepper, corn, and black beans.
4. Top the salad with the cooked turkey mixture.
5. Sprinkle with shredded cheddar cheese, and arrange avocado slices on top.
6. Drizzle with salsa and serve immediately.

Nutrition Info per Serving (Serves 4):

- Calories: 350
- Protein: 28g
- Carbohydrates: 20g
- Dietary Fiber: 8g
- Sugars: 5g
- Total Fat: 18g
- Saturated Fat: 4g
- Sodium: 320mg

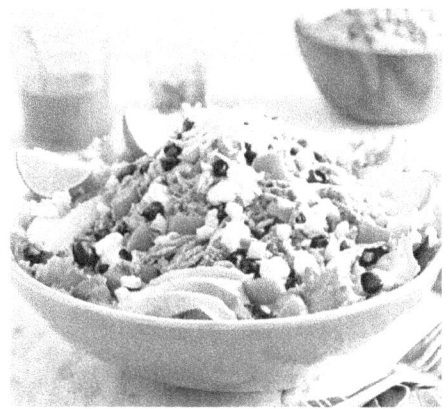

Servings: 4 Cooking Time: 20 minutes

22. Stuffed Turkey Breast with Spinach and Walnuts

Ingredients:

- 1 pound turkey breast, butterflied
- 1 tablespoon olive oil
- 1 cup fresh spinach, chopped
- 1/4 cup walnuts, chopped
- 1/4 cup crumbled feta cheese
- 2 cloves garlic, minced
- 1 teaspoon dried thyme
- 1/4 teaspoon ground black pepper

Instructions:

1. Preheat the oven to 375°F (190°C).
2. In a skillet, heat the olive oil over medium heat. Add the minced garlic and cook until fragrant, about 1 minute.
3. Add the chopped spinach and cook until wilted, about 2-3 minutes. Remove from heat and stir in the chopped walnuts and crumbled feta cheese.
4. Spread the spinach mixture over the butterflied turkey breast. Roll up the turkey breast and secure with kitchen twine.
5. Place the stuffed turkey breast in a baking dish. Sprinkle with dried thyme and black pepper.
6. Bake for 35-40 minutes, or until the turkey is cooked through and reaches an internal temperature of 165°F (75°C).
7. Let the turkey rest for 5 minutes before slicing and serving.

Nutrition Info per Serving (Serves 4):

- Calories: 300
- Protein: 30g
- Carbohydrates: 5g
- Dietary Fiber: 2g
- Sugars: 1g
- Total Fat: 18g
- Saturated Fat: 4g
- Sodium: 200mg

Servings: 4 Cooking Time: 45 minutes

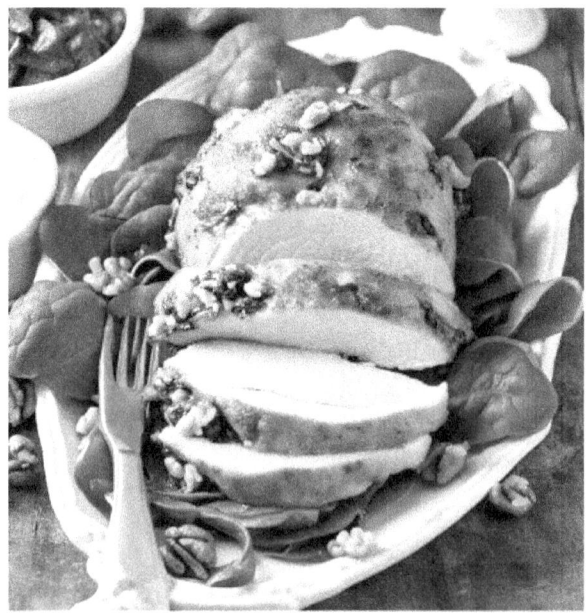

23. Turkey Picadillo

Ingredients:

- 1 pound ground turkey
- 2 tablespoons olive oil
- 1 onion, chopped
- 2 cloves garlic, minced
- 1 red bell pepper, chopped
- 1 can (14.5 oz) diced tomatoes, no salt added
- 1/4 cup green olives, sliced
- 1/4 cup raisins
- 1 tablespoon ground cumin
- 1 teaspoon paprika
- 1 teaspoon dried oregano
- 1/4 teaspoon ground black pepper

Instructions:

1. Heat the olive oil in a large skillet over medium-high heat. Add the ground turkey and cook until browned, about 5-7 minutes.
2. Add the chopped onion, garlic, and red bell pepper. Cook until softened, about 5 minutes.
3. Stir in the diced tomatoes, green olives, raisins, cumin, paprika, oregano, and black pepper.
4. Reduce the heat and simmer for 15-20 minutes, until the flavors meld together.
5. Serve hot.

Nutrition Info per Serving (Serves 4):

- Calories: 300
- Protein: 28g
- Carbohydrates: 18g
- Dietary Fiber: 4g
- Sugars: 10g
- Total Fat: 14g
- Saturated Fat: 2g
- Sodium: 380mg

Servings: 4 Cooking Time: 30 minutes

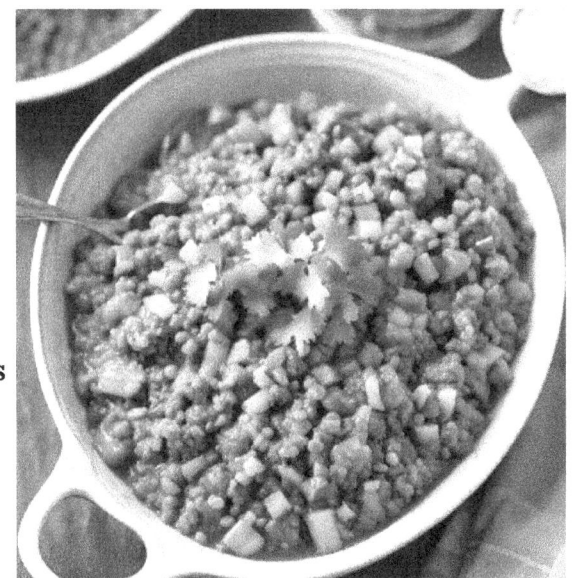

24. Herb Roasted Turkey Thighs

Ingredients:

- 4 turkey thighs
- 2 tablespoons olive oil
- 1 tablespoon dried rosemary
- 1 tablespoon dried thyme
- 1 teaspoon garlic powder
- 1/4 teaspoon ground black pepper
- 1 lemon, sliced

Instructions:

1. Preheat the oven to 375°F (190°C).
2. In a small bowl, mix the olive oil, rosemary, thyme, garlic powder, and black pepper.
3. Rub the herb mixture all over the turkey thighs.
4. Place the turkey thighs in a baking dish and arrange the lemon slices on top.
5. Roast in the preheated oven for 45-50 minutes, or until the turkey thighs reach an internal temperature of 165°F (75°C).
6. Let rest for 5 minutes before serving.

Nutrition Info per Serving (Serves 4):

- Calories: 400
- Protein: 40g
- Carbohydrates: 3g
- Dietary Fiber: 1g
- Sugars: 1g
- Total Fat: 25g
- Saturated Fat: 6g
- Sodium: 150mg

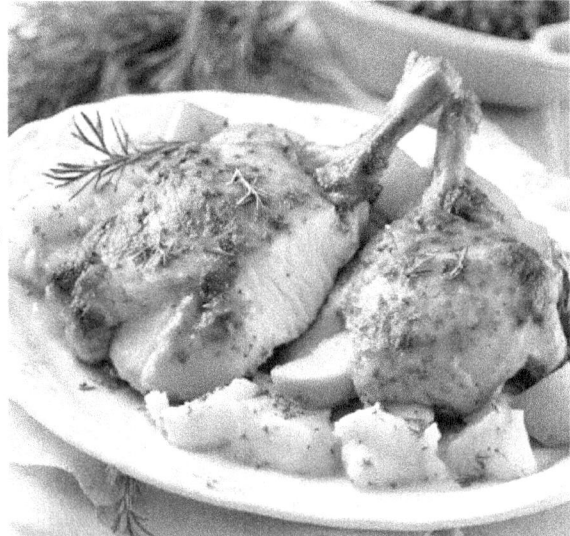

Servings: 4 Cooking Time: 50 minutes

25. Turkey Stew with Root Vegetables

Ingredients:

- 1 pound turkey breast, cubed
- 2 tablespoons olive oil
- 1 onion, chopped
- 2 cloves garlic, minced
- 2 carrots, sliced
- 2 parsnips, sliced
- 2 potatoes, cubed
- 4 cups low-sodium chicken broth
- 1 teaspoon dried thyme
- 1 teaspoon dried rosemary
- 1/4 teaspoon ground black pepper

Instructions:

1. Heat the olive oil in a large pot over medium-high heat. Add the cubed turkey and cook until browned, about 5-7 minutes. Remove and set aside.
2. In the same pot, add the chopped onion and garlic. Cook until softened, about 3-4 minutes.
3. Add the carrots, parsnips, and potatoes. Cook for another 5 minutes, stirring occasionally.
4. Pour in the chicken broth, and add the thyme, rosemary, and black pepper.
5. Return the turkey to the pot and bring to a boil. Reduce the heat and simmer for 30 minutes, or until the vegetables are tender and the stew has thickened.
6. Serve hot.

Nutrition Info per Serving (Serves 4):

- Calories: 350
- Protein: 30g
- Carbohydrates: 30g
- Dietary Fiber: 6g
- Sugars: 6g
- Total Fat: 12g
- Saturated Fat: 2g
- Sodium: 300mg

Servings: 4 Cooking Time: 45 minutes

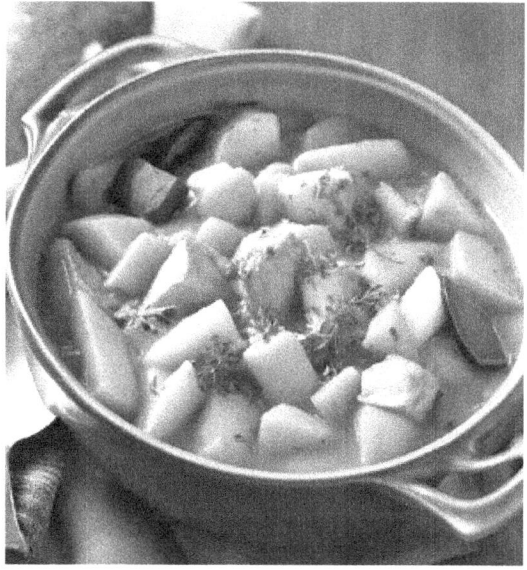

26. Turkey and Cranberry Salad

Ingredients:
- 2 cups cooked turkey breast, chopped
- 4 cups mixed salad greens
- 1/2 cup dried cranberries
- 1/4 cup walnuts, chopped
- 1/4 cup crumbled feta cheese
- 1 apple, cored and sliced
- 2 tablespoons olive oil
- 1 tablespoon balsamic vinegar
- 1 teaspoon Dijon mustard
- 1/4 teaspoon ground black pepper

Instructions:
1. In a large bowl, combine the cooked turkey, salad greens, dried cranberries, walnuts, feta cheese, and apple slices.
2. In a small bowl, whisk together the olive oil, balsamic vinegar, Dijon mustard, and black pepper.
3. Drizzle the dressing over the salad and toss to combine.
4. Serve immediately.

Nutrition Info per Serving (Serves 4):
- Calories: 320
- Protein: 24g
- Carbohydrates: 20g
- Dietary Fiber: 4g
- Sugars: 12g
- Total Fat: 16g
- Saturated Fat: 4g
- Sodium: 220mg

Servings: 4 Cooking Time: 10 minutes

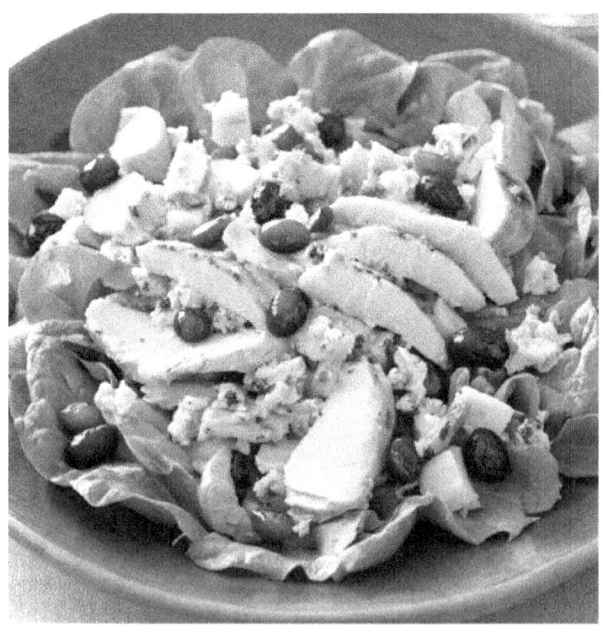

Fish and Seafood Recipes

1. Grilled Salmon with Dill Yogurt Sauce
Ingredients:
- 4 salmon fillets (about 6 ounces each)
- 2 tablespoons olive oil
- 1 teaspoon garlic powder
- 1 teaspoon dried dill
- 1 cup plain Greek yogurt
- 1 tablespoon fresh dill, chopped
- 1 tablespoon lemon juice
- 1 teaspoon Dijon mustard
- 1/4 teaspoon ground black pepper

Instructions:
1. Preheat the grill to medium-high heat.
2. Brush the salmon fillets with olive oil and sprinkle with garlic powder and dried dill.
3. Grill the salmon fillets for 4-5 minutes per side, or until the salmon is cooked through and flakes easily with a fork.
4. While the salmon is grilling, prepare the dill yogurt sauce. In a small bowl, combine the Greek yogurt, fresh dill, lemon juice, Dijon mustard, and black pepper. Mix well.
5. Serve the grilled salmon fillets topped with the dill yogurt sauce.

Nutrition Info per Serving (Serves 4):
- Calories: 350
- Protein: 34g
- Carbohydrates: 5g
- Dietary Fiber: 0g
- Sugars: 3g
- Total Fat: 22g
- Saturated Fat: 4g
- Sodium: 180mg

Servings: 4 Cooking Time: 15 minutes

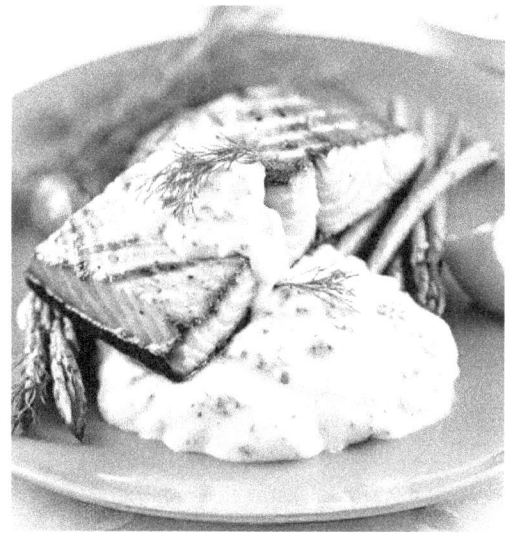

2. Turkey Veggie Pasta

Ingredients:

- 1 pound ground turkey
- 2 tablespoons olive oil
- 1 onion, chopped
- 2 cloves garlic, minced
- 1 red bell pepper, chopped
- 1 zucchini, chopped
- 1 can (14.5 oz) diced tomatoes, no salt added
- 1 teaspoon dried basil
- 1 teaspoon dried oregano
- 1/4 teaspoon ground black pepper
- 8 ounces whole wheat pasta

Instructions:

1. Cook the whole wheat pasta according to the package instructions. Drain and set aside.
2. In a large skillet, heat the olive oil over medium-high heat. Add the ground turkey and cook until browned, about 5-7 minutes.
3. Add the chopped onion, garlic, red bell pepper, and zucchini. Cook until the vegetables are tender, about 5 minutes.
4. Stir in the diced tomatoes, dried basil, oregano, and black pepper. Simmer for 10 minutes.
5. Toss the cooked pasta with the turkey and vegetable mixture. Serve immediately.

Nutrition Info per Serving (Serves 4):

- Calories: 400
- Protein: 30g
- Carbohydrates: 45g
- Dietary Fiber: 8g
- Sugars: 7g
- Total Fat: 12g
- Saturated Fat: 2g
- Sodium: 180mg

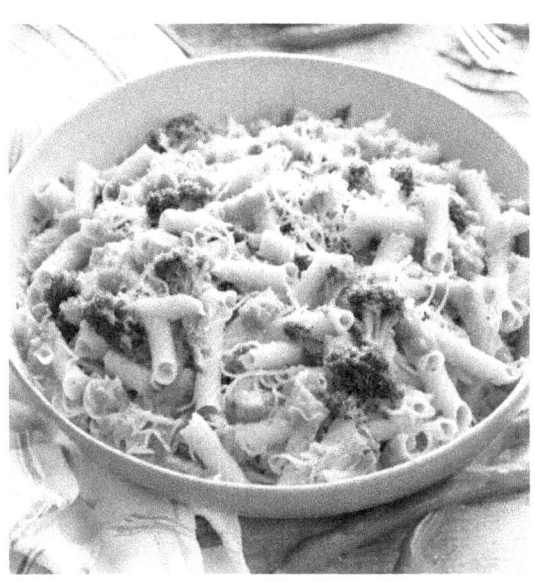

Servings: 4 Cooking Time: 25 minutes

3. Baked Cod with Lemon and Capers

Ingredients:
- 4 cod fillets (about 6 ounces each)
- 2 tablespoons olive oil
- 1 lemon, thinly sliced
- 2 tablespoons capers, rinsed and drained
- 1 teaspoon garlic powder
- 1 teaspoon dried thyme
- 1/4 teaspoon ground black pepper

Instructions:
1. Preheat the oven to 400°F (200°C).
2. Place the cod fillets in a baking dish. Drizzle with olive oil and sprinkle with garlic powder, dried thyme, and black pepper.
3. Arrange the lemon slices on top of the cod fillets and scatter the capers over the top.
4. Bake for 15-20 minutes, or until the cod is cooked through and flakes easily with a fork.
5. Serve immediately.

Nutrition Info per Serving (Serves 4):
- Calories: 200
- Protein: 30g
- Carbohydrates: 2g
- Dietary Fiber: 0g
- Sugars: 0g
- Total Fat: 8g
- Saturated Fat: 1g
- Sodium: 200mg

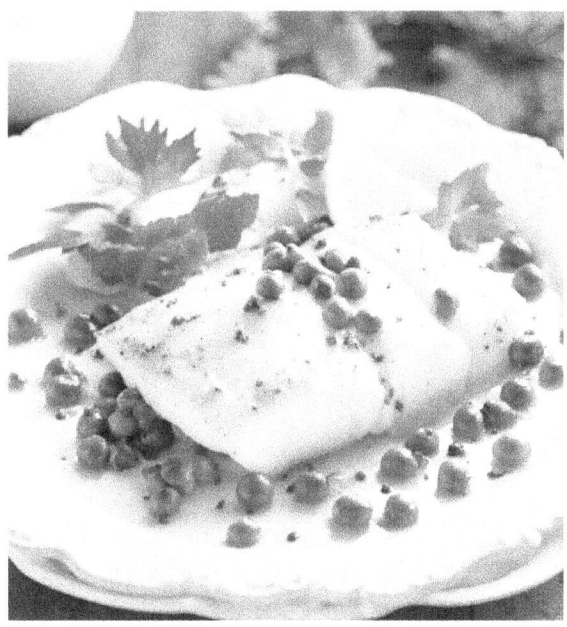

Servings: 4 Cooking Time: 20 minutes

4. Tuna Salad with White Beans

Ingredients:

- 2 cans (5 oz each) tuna packed in water, drained
- 1 can (15 oz) white beans, drained and rinsed
- 1/2 cup red onion, finely chopped
- 1/2 cup celery, finely chopped
- 1/4 cup fresh parsley, chopped
- 2 tablespoons olive oil
- 1 tablespoon lemon juice
- 1 teaspoon Dijon mustard
- 1/4 teaspoon ground black pepper

Instructions:

1. In a large bowl, combine the drained tuna, white beans, red onion, celery, and parsley.
2. In a small bowl, whisk together the olive oil, lemon juice, Dijon mustard, and black pepper.
3. Pour the dressing over the tuna mixture and toss to combine.
4. Serve immediately or refrigerate until ready to serve.

Nutrition Info per Serving (Serves 4):

- Calories: 250
- Protein: 25g
- Carbohydrates: 20g
- Dietary Fiber: 6g
- Sugars: 2g
- Total Fat: 10g
- Saturated Fat: 1.5g
- Sodium: 220mg

Servings: 4 Cooking Time: 10 minutes

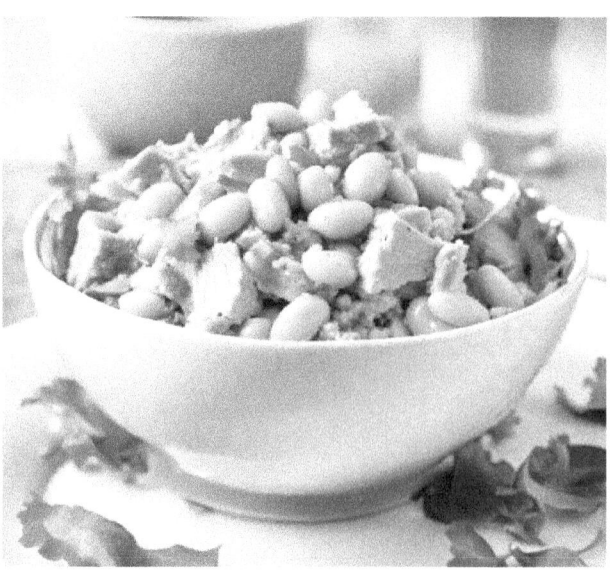

5. Pan-Seared Trout with Almonds
Ingredients:
- 4 trout fillets (about 6 ounces each)
- 2 tablespoons olive oil
- 1/4 cup sliced almonds
- 2 cloves garlic, minced
- 1 lemon, juiced
- 1 tablespoon fresh parsley, chopped
- 1/4 teaspoon ground black pepper

Instructions:
1. Heat 1 tablespoon of olive oil in a large skillet over medium-high heat.
2. Add the trout fillets to the skillet, skin side down, and cook for 4-5 minutes per side, until the fish is cooked through and flakes easily with a fork. Remove from the skillet and set aside.
3. In the same skillet, add the remaining olive oil and sliced almonds. Cook for 2-3 minutes, stirring frequently, until the almonds are golden brown.
4. Add the minced garlic and cook for an additional 1 minute until fragrant.
5. Remove the skillet from heat and stir in the lemon juice and black pepper.
6. Spoon the almond mixture over the trout fillets and sprinkle with chopped parsley.
7. Serve immediately.

Nutrition Info per Serving (Serves 4):
- Calories: 320
- Protein: 32g
- Carbohydrates: 4g
- Dietary Fiber: 1g
- Sugars: 0g
- Total Fat: 20g
- Saturated Fat: 3g
- Sodium: 100mg

Servings: 4 Cooking Time: 15 minutes

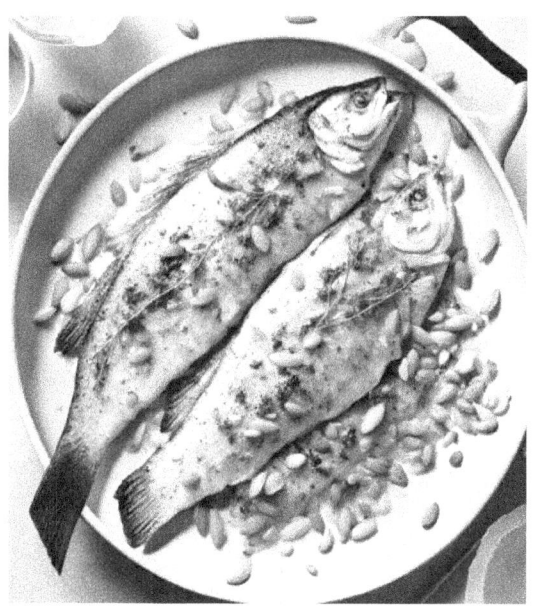

6. Herb-Baked Tilapia

Ingredients:

- 4 tilapia fillets (about 6 ounces each)
- 2 tablespoons olive oil
- 1 teaspoon dried thyme
- 1 teaspoon dried basil
- 1 teaspoon garlic powder
- 1 lemon, thinly sliced
- 1/4 teaspoon ground black pepper

Instructions:

1. Preheat the oven to 375°F (190°C).
2. Place the tilapia fillets in a baking dish. Drizzle with olive oil and sprinkle with thyme, basil, garlic powder, and black pepper.
3. Arrange the lemon slices on top of the fillets.
4. Bake for 15-20 minutes, or until the tilapia is cooked through and flakes easily with a fork.
5. Serve immediately.

Nutrition Info per Serving (Serves 4):

- Calories: 220
- Protein: 28g
- Carbohydrates: 2g
- Dietary Fiber: 1g
- Sugars: 0g
- Total Fat: 10g
- Saturated Fat: 2g
- Sodium: 100mg

Servings: 4 Cooking Time: 20 minutes

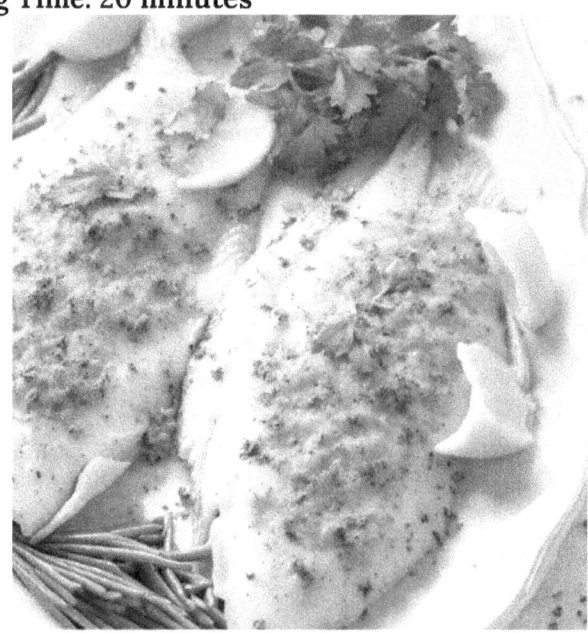

7. Sardines on Toast

Ingredients:

- 4 slices whole grain bread
- 2 cans (3.75 oz each) sardines in olive oil, drained
- 1/2 lemon, juiced
- 1 tablespoon fresh parsley, chopped
- 1/4 teaspoon ground black pepper

Instructions:

1. Toast the whole grain bread slices until golden brown.
2. In a bowl, combine the sardines, lemon juice, parsley, and black pepper. Mix well, breaking up the sardines with a fork.
3. Spread the sardine mixture evenly over the toasted bread slices.
4. Serve immediately.

Nutrition Info per Serving (Serves 4):

- Calories: 200
- Protein: 14g
- Carbohydrates: 20g
- Dietary Fiber: 4g
- Sugars: 1g
- Total Fat: 9g
- Saturated Fat: 2g
- Sodium: 180mg

Servings: 4 Cooking Time: 10 minutes

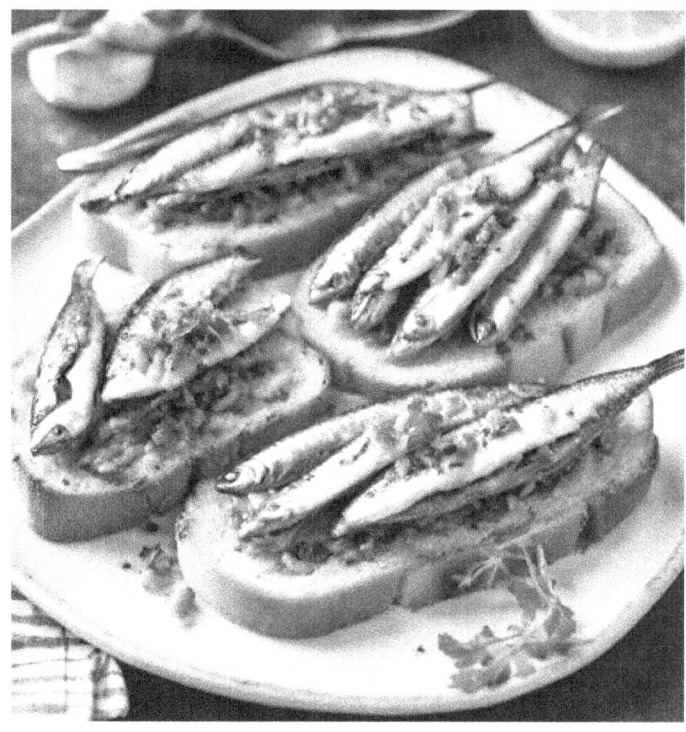

8. Mackerel Salad

Ingredients:

- 2 cups cooked mackerel, flaked
- 4 cups mixed salad greens
- 1/2 cup cherry tomatoes, halved
- 1/4 cup red onion, thinly sliced
- 1/4 cup kalamata olives, pitted and sliced
- 1/4 cup crumbled feta cheese
- 2 tablespoons olive oil
- 1 tablespoon lemon juice
- 1 teaspoon Dijon mustard
- 1/4 teaspoon ground black pepper

Instructions:

1. In a large bowl, combine the flaked mackerel, mixed salad greens, cherry tomatoes, red onion, olives, and feta cheese.
2. In a small bowl, whisk together the olive oil, lemon juice, Dijon mustard, and black pepper.
3. Drizzle the dressing over the salad and toss to combine.
4. Serve immediately.

Nutrition Info per Serving (Serves 4):

- Calories: 280
- Protein: 20g
- Carbohydrates: 6g
- Dietary Fiber: 2g
- Sugars: 3g
- Total Fat: 20g
- Saturated Fat: 4g
- Sodium: 300mg

Servings: 4 Cooking Time: 10 minute

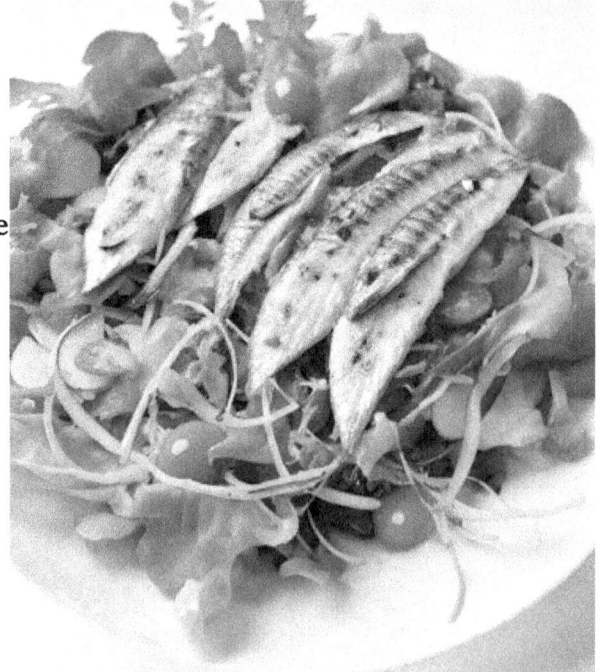

9. Pesto Salmon Skewers

Ingredients:

- 1 pound salmon fillet, cut into cubes
- 2 tablespoons olive oil
- 1/4 cup basil pesto
- 1 red bell pepper, cut into squares
- 1 yellow bell pepper, cut into squares
- 1 red onion, cut into squares
- 1/4 teaspoon ground black pepper

Instructions:

1. Preheat the grill to medium-high heat.
2. In a bowl, toss the salmon cubes with olive oil, basil pesto, and black pepper.
3. Thread the salmon, red bell pepper, yellow bell pepper, and red onion onto skewers.
4. Grill the skewers for 8-10 minutes, turning occasionally, until the salmon is cooked through and the vegetables are tender.
5. Serve immediately.

Nutrition Info per Serving (Serves 4):

- Calories: 320
- Protein: 25g
- Carbohydrates: 6g
- Dietary Fiber: 2g
- Sugars: 3g
- Total Fat: 22g
- Saturated Fat: 4g
- Sodium: 200mg

Servings: 4 Cooking Time: 15 minutes

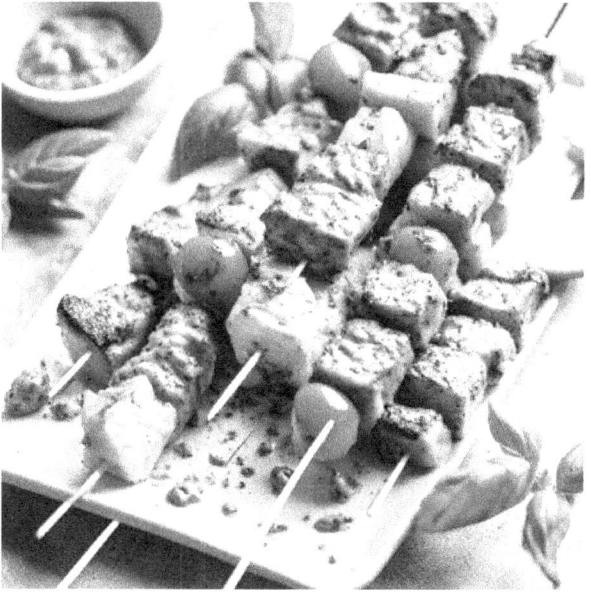

10. Haddock in Tomato Basil Sauce

Ingredients:

- 4 haddock fillets (about 6 ounces each)
- 2 tablespoons olive oil
- 1 onion, chopped
- 2 cloves garlic, minced
- 1 can (14.5 oz) diced tomatoes, no salt added
- 1/4 cup fresh basil, chopped
- 1 teaspoon dried oregano
- 1/4 teaspoon ground black pepper

Instructions:

1. Preheat the oven to 375°F (190°C).
2. In a skillet, heat the olive oil over medium heat. Add the chopped onion and garlic, and sauté until softened, about 3-4 minutes.
3. Stir in the diced tomatoes, fresh basil, dried oregano, and black pepper. Simmer for 10 minutes.
4. Place the haddock fillets in a baking dish and pour the tomato basil sauce over the top.
5. Bake for 20-25 minutes, or until the haddock is cooked through and flakes easily with a fork.
6. Serve immediately.

Nutrition Info per Serving (Serves 4):

- Calories: 230
- Protein: 32g
- Carbohydrates: 8g
- Dietary Fiber: 2g
- Sugars: 4g
- Total Fat: 8g
- Saturated Fat: 1.5g
- Sodium: 220mg

Servings: 4 Cooking Time: 35 minutes

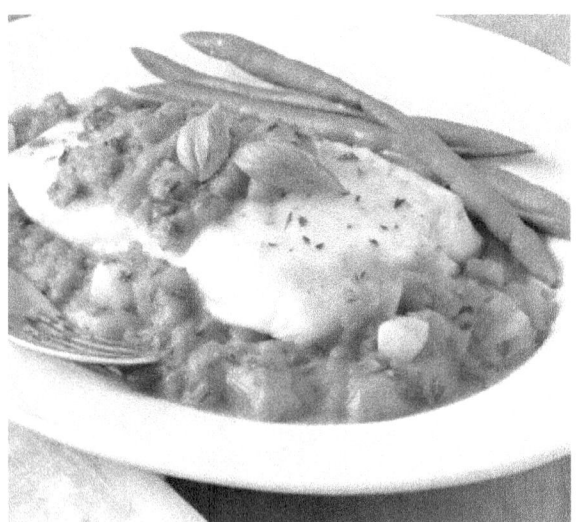

11. Lemon Garlic Halibut

Ingredients:

- 4 halibut fillets (about 6 ounces each)
- 2 tablespoons olive oil
- 2 cloves garlic, minced
- 1 lemon, thinly sliced
- 1/4 cup fresh parsley, chopped
- 1/4 teaspoon ground black pepper

Instructions:

1. Preheat the oven to 375°F (190°C).
2. Place the halibut fillets in a baking dish.
3. In a small bowl, mix the olive oil and minced garlic. Brush the mixture over the halibut fillets.
4. Arrange the lemon slices on top of the fillets.
5. Bake for 15-20 minutes, or until the halibut is cooked through and flakes easily with a fork.
6. Sprinkle with chopped parsley and ground black pepper before serving.

Nutrition Info per Serving (Serves 4):

- Calories: 230
- Protein: 35g
- Carbohydrates: 2g
- Dietary Fiber: 1g
- Sugars: 0g
- Total Fat: 10g
- Saturated Fat: 2g
- Sodium: 80mg

Servings: 4 Cooking Time: 20 minutes

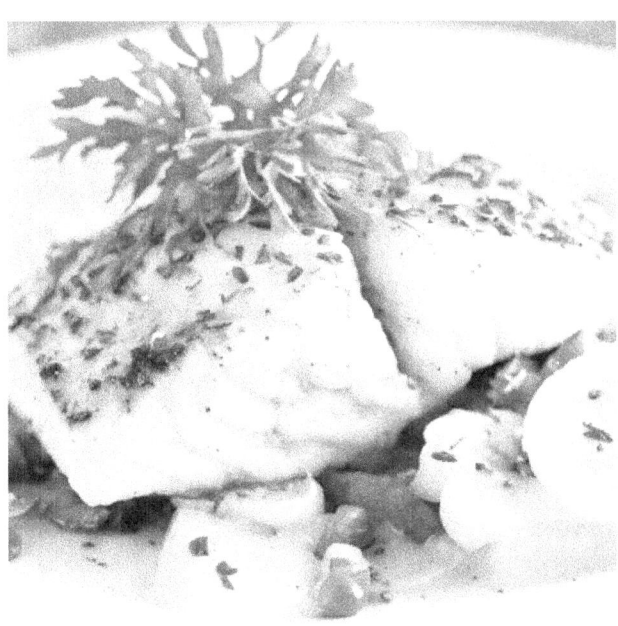

12. Sole Meunière

Ingredients:

- 4 sole fillets (about 6 ounces each)
- 1/4 cup whole wheat flour
- 2 tablespoons olive oil
- 1 lemon, juiced
- 2 tablespoons fresh parsley, chopped
- 1/4 teaspoon ground black pepper

Instructions:

1. Lightly coat the sole fillets in whole wheat flour, shaking off any excess.
2. Heat the olive oil in a large skillet over medium-high heat.
3. Add the sole fillets and cook for 2-3 minutes on each side, until golden brown and cooked through.
4. Remove the fish from the skillet and place on a serving platter.
5. Pour the lemon juice into the skillet and let it simmer for 1 minute, scraping up any browned bits from the bottom of the pan.
6. Pour the lemon sauce over the fish and sprinkle with chopped parsley and ground black pepper.
7. Serve immediately.

Nutrition Info per Serving (Serves 4):

- Calories: 220
- Protein: 30g
- Carbohydrates: 6g
- Dietary Fiber: 1g
- Sugars: 1g
- Total Fat: 9g
- Saturated Fat: 1.5g
- Sodium: 100mg

Servings: 4 Cooking Time: 15 minutes

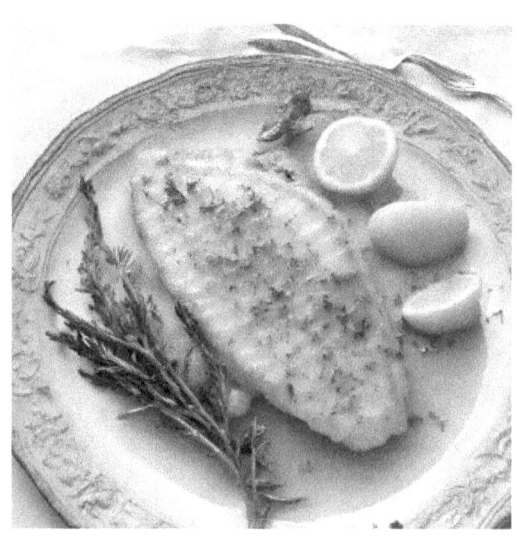

13. Curried Shrimp and Quinoa Salad

Ingredients:

- 1 cup quinoa
- 2 cups water
- 1 pound shrimp, peeled and deveined
- 2 tablespoons olive oil, divided
- 1 tablespoon curry powder
- 1 red bell pepper, chopped
- 1 cucumber, chopped
- 1/4 cup red onion, finely chopped
- 1/4 cup fresh cilantro, chopped
- 1 tablespoon lemon juice
- 1/4 teaspoon ground black pepper

Instructions:

1. Rinse the quinoa under cold water. In a medium saucepan, bring the water to a boil. Add the quinoa, reduce heat to low, cover, and simmer for 15 minutes or until the water is absorbed and the quinoa is tender. Let cool.
2. In a large skillet, heat 1 tablespoon of olive oil over medium-high heat. Add the shrimp and curry powder, and cook for 3-4 minutes until the shrimp is pink and opaque. Remove from heat and let cool.
3. In a large bowl, combine the cooked quinoa, shrimp, red bell pepper, cucumber, red onion, and cilantro.
4. In a small bowl, whisk together the remaining olive oil, lemon juice, and black pepper. Pour over the salad and toss to combine.
5. Serve immediately or refrigerate until ready to serve.

Nutrition Info per Serving (Serves 4):

- Calories: 350
- Protein: 28g
- Carbohydrates: 28g
- Dietary Fiber: 5g
- Sugars: 4g
- Total Fat: 14g
- Saturated Fat: 2g
- Sodium: 200mg

Servings: 4 Cooking Time: 25 minutes

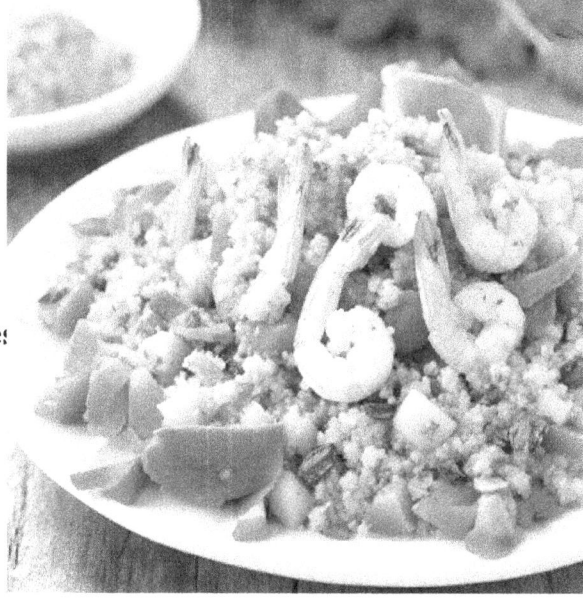

14. Grilled Mackerel with Salsa Verde

Ingredients:

- 4 mackerel fillets (about 6 ounces each)
- 2 tablespoons olive oil
- 1 lemon, juiced
- 1 cup fresh parsley, chopped
- 1/2 cup fresh cilantro, chopped
- 1/4 cup capers, rinsed and drained
- 2 cloves garlic, minced
- 1/4 teaspoon ground black pepper

Instructions:

1. Preheat the grill to medium-high heat.
2. Brush the mackerel fillets with 1 tablespoon of olive oil and grill for 4-5 minutes on each side, until the fish is cooked through and flakes easily with a fork.
3. While the fish is grilling, prepare the salsa verde by combining the parsley, cilantro, capers, garlic, lemon juice, remaining olive oil, and black pepper in a bowl. Mix well.
4. Serve the grilled mackerel topped with the salsa verde.

Nutrition Info per Serving (Serves 4):

- Calories: 310
- Protein: 28g
- Carbohydrates: 3g
- Dietary Fiber: 1g
- Sugars: 0g
- Total Fat: 20g
- Saturated Fat: 4g
- Sodium: 150mg

Servings: 4 Cooking Time: 15 minutes

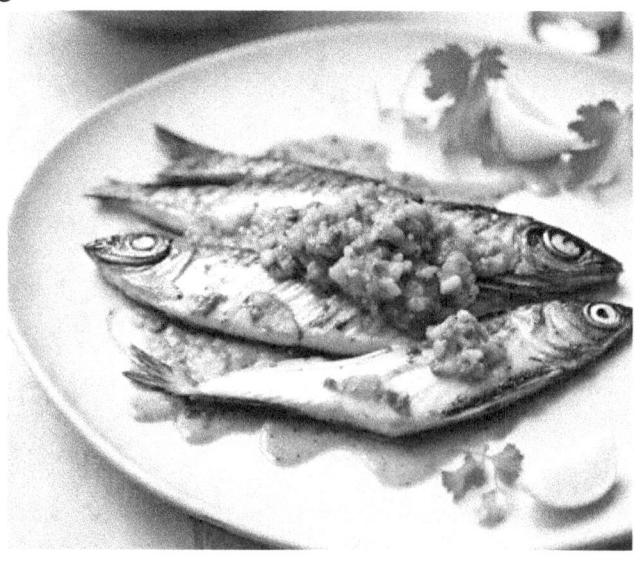

15. Baked Sardines with Herbs

Ingredients:

- 12 fresh sardines, cleaned and gutted
- 3 tablespoons olive oil
- 1 lemon, sliced
- 2 cloves garlic, minced
- 1 tablespoon fresh thyme, chopped
- 1 tablespoon fresh rosemary, chopped
- 1/4 teaspoon ground black pepper

Instructions:

1. Preheat the oven to 400°F (200°C).
2. Arrange the sardines in a single layer on a baking sheet.
3. Drizzle with olive oil and sprinkle with garlic, thyme, rosemary, and black pepper.
4. Arrange the lemon slices over the sardines.
5. Bake for 15-20 minutes, or until the sardines are cooked through and the skin is crispy.
6. Serve immediately.

Nutrition Info per Serving (Serves 4):

- Calories: 250
- Protein: 26g
- Carbohydrates: 2g
- Dietary Fiber: 1g
- Sugars: 0g
- Total Fat: 16g
- Saturated Fat: 3g
- Sodium: 120mg

Servings: 4 Cooking Time: 20 minutes

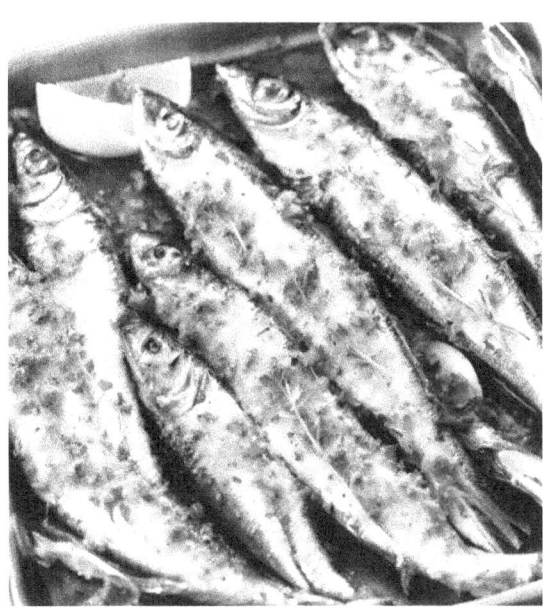

16. Fish Stew with Tomatoes and Olives

Ingredients:

- 1 pound white fish fillets (such as cod or halibut), cut into chunks
- 2 tablespoons olive oil
- 1 onion, chopped
- 2 cloves garlic, minced
- 1 can (14.5 oz) diced tomatoes, no salt added
- 1 cup low-sodium chicken broth
- 1/2 cup green olives, pitted and sliced
- 1/4 cup fresh parsley, chopped
- 1 teaspoon dried thyme
- 1/4 teaspoon ground black pepper

Instructions:

1. In a large pot, heat the olive oil over medium heat. Add the chopped onion and minced garlic, and sauté until softened, about 3-4 minutes.
2. Stir in the diced tomatoes, chicken broth, olives, thyme, and black pepper. Bring to a boil, then reduce the heat and simmer for 10 minutes.
3. Add the fish chunks to the pot and simmer for another 5-7 minutes, or until the fish is cooked through and flakes easily.
4. Stir in the chopped parsley and serve hot.

Nutrition Info per Serving (Serves 4):

- Calories: 220
- Protein: 30g
- Carbohydrates: 8g
- Dietary Fiber: 2g
- Sugars: 4g
- Total Fat: 8g
- Saturated Fat: 1.5g
- Sodium: 200mg

Servings: 4 Cooking Time: 25 minutes

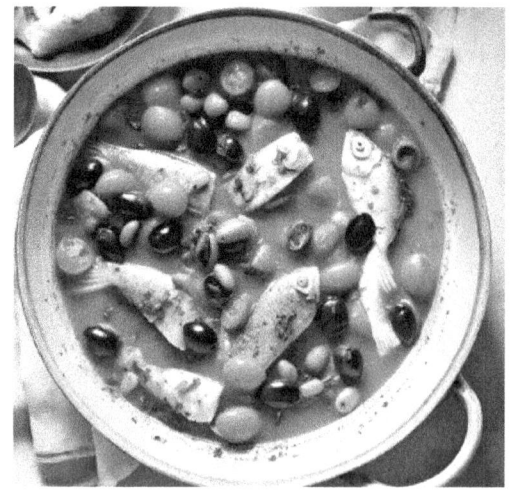

17. Roasted Trout with Fennel

Ingredients:
- 4 trout fillets (about 6 ounces each)
- 2 tablespoons olive oil
- 1 fennel bulb, thinly sliced
- 2 cloves garlic, minced
- 1 lemon, sliced
- 1/4 cup fresh dill, chopped
- 1/4 teaspoon ground black pepper

Instructions:
1. Preheat the oven to 375°F (190°C).
2. Place the trout fillets on a baking sheet.
3. In a bowl, combine the olive oil, minced garlic, and black pepper. Brush the mixture over the trout fillets.
4. Arrange the fennel slices and lemon slices over and around the trout.
5. Roast in the oven for 20-25 minutes, or until the trout is cooked through and flakes easily with a fork.
6. Sprinkle with chopped dill before serving.

Nutrition Info per Serving (Serves 4):
- Calories: 290
- Protein: 30g
- Carbohydrates: 5g
- Dietary Fiber: 1g
- Sugars: 1g
- Total Fat: 17g
- Saturated Fat: 3g
- Sodium: 100mg

Servings: 4 Cooking Time: 30 minutes

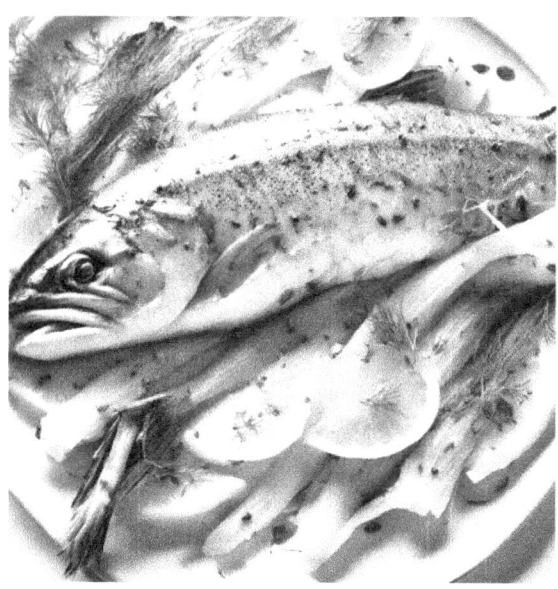

18. Salmon Patties with Lemon Aioli

Ingredients:

- 1 pound cooked salmon, flaked
- 1/2 cup whole wheat breadcrumbs
- 1/4 cup finely chopped red onion
- 2 cloves garlic, minced
- 1/4 cup fresh parsley, chopped
- 2 large eggs, beaten
- 2 tablespoons olive oil
- 1/4 teaspoon ground black pepper

Lemon Aioli:

- 1/2 cup plain Greek yogurt
- 1 tablespoon lemon juice
- 1 teaspoon lemon zest
- 1 clove garlic, minced

Instructions:

1. In a large bowl, combine the flaked salmon, breadcrumbs, red onion, garlic, parsley, eggs, and black pepper. Mix well and form into 8 patties.
2. Heat the olive oil in a large skillet over medium heat. Cook the salmon patties for 3-4 minutes on each side, until golden brown and heated through.
3. To make the lemon aioli, mix the Greek yogurt, lemon juice, lemon zest, and garlic in a small bowl.
4. Serve the salmon patties with a dollop of lemon aioli.

Nutrition Info per Serving (Serves 4):

- Calories: 320
- Protein: 28g
- Carbohydrates: 14g
- Dietary Fiber: 2g
- Sugars: 3g
- Total Fat: 18g
- Saturated Fat: 3g
- Sodium: 220mg

Servings: 4 Cooking Time: 20 minutes

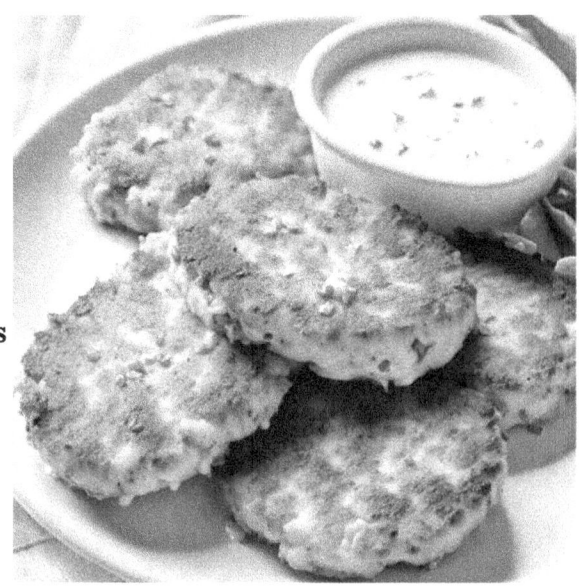

19. Flounder with Parsley and Garlic

Ingredients:

- 4 flounder fillets (about 6 ounces each)
- 2 tablespoons olive oil
- 3 cloves garlic, minced
- 1/4 cup fresh parsley, chopped
- 1 lemon, juiced
- 1/4 teaspoon ground black pepper

Instructions:

1. Preheat the oven to 375°F (190°C).
2. Place the flounder fillets in a baking dish.
3. In a small bowl, mix the olive oil, garlic, parsley, lemon juice, and black pepper. Pour the mixture over the flounder fillets.
4. Bake for 15-20 minutes, or until the fish is cooked through and flakes easily with a fork.
5. Serve immediately.

Nutrition Info per Serving (Serves 4):

- Calories: 240
- Protein: 30g
- Carbohydrates: 4g
- Dietary Fiber: 1g
- Sugars: 1g
- Total Fat: 12g
- Saturated Fat: 2g
- Sodium: 100mg

Servings: 4 Cooking Time: 20 minutes

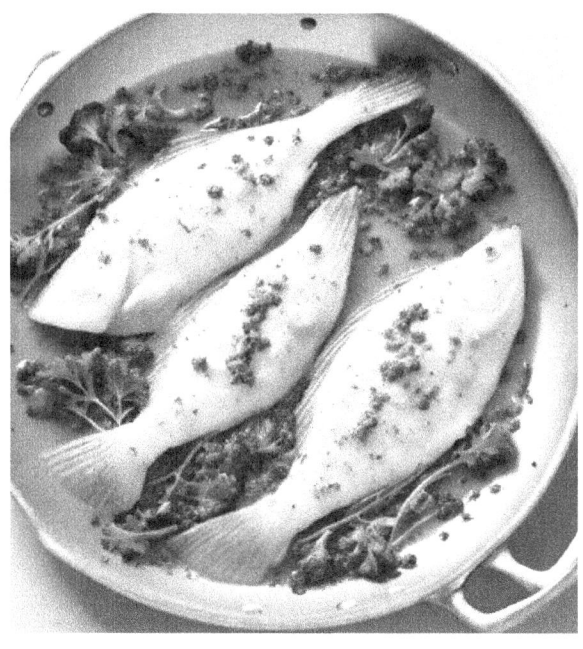

20. Grilled Calamari with Olive Oil and Lemon

Ingredients:

- 1 pound calamari, cleaned and cut into rings
- 3 tablespoons olive oil
- 2 cloves garlic, minced
- 1 lemon, juiced
- 1/4 cup fresh parsley, chopped
- 1/4 teaspoon ground black pepper

Instructions:

1. Preheat the grill to medium-high heat.
2. In a bowl, toss the calamari rings with 2 tablespoons of olive oil, garlic, and black pepper.
3. Grill the calamari for 2-3 minutes on each side, until opaque and slightly charred.
4. In a small bowl, mix the remaining olive oil, lemon juice, and parsley.
5. Drizzle the lemon and parsley mixture over the grilled calamari before serving.

Nutrition Info per Serving (Serves 4):

- Calories: 200
- Protein: 26g
- Carbohydrates: 3g
- Dietary Fiber: 1g
- Sugars: 0g
- Total Fat: 10g
- Saturated Fat: 1.5g
- Sodium: 150mg

Servings: 4 Cooking Time: 10 minutes

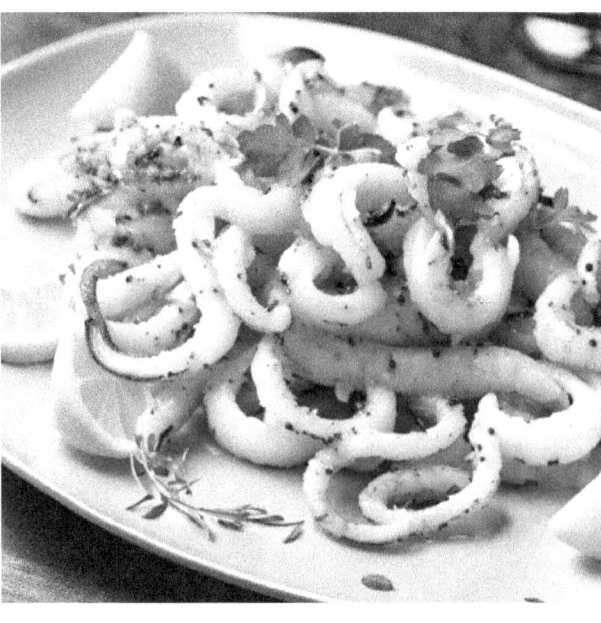

21. Shrimp Caesar Salad

Ingredients:
- 1 pound shrimp, peeled and deveined
- 2 tablespoons olive oil
- 1/2 teaspoon garlic powder
- 1/4 teaspoon ground black pepper
- 4 cups romaine lettuce, chopped
- 1/4 cup grated Parmesan cheese
- 1/4 cup whole wheat croutons

Caesar Dressing:
- 1/2 cup plain Greek yogurt
- 1 tablespoon lemon juice
- 1 teaspoon Dijon mustard
- 2 cloves garlic, minced
- 1 teaspoon Worcestershire sauce

Instructions:
1. Preheat the oven to 400°F (200°C).
2. Toss the shrimp with olive oil, garlic powder, and black pepper. Spread the shrimp on a baking sheet and roast for 8-10 minutes, or until pink and cooked through.
3. In a small bowl, whisk together the Greek yogurt, lemon juice, Dijon mustard, minced garlic, and Worcestershire sauce to make the Caesar dressing.
4. In a large bowl, combine the chopped romaine lettuce, roasted shrimp, Parmesan cheese, and croutons.
5. Drizzle the Caesar dressing over the salad and toss to combine.
6. Serve immediately.

Nutrition Info per Serving (Serves 4):
- Calories: 280
- Protein: 30g
- Carbohydrates: 10g
- Dietary Fiber: 2g
- Sugars: 3g
- Total Fat: 14g
- Saturated Fat: 3g
- Sodium: 400mg

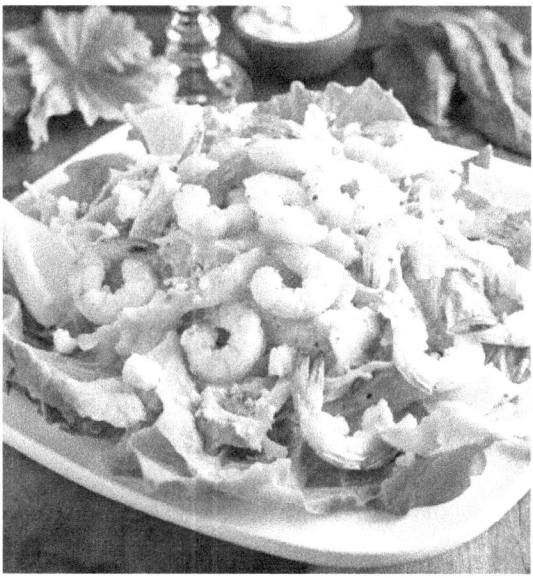

Servings: 4 Cooking Time: 15 minutes

22. Lobster Thermidor

Ingredients:

- 2 lobster tails, cooked and meat chopped
- 2 tablespoons olive oil
- 1 small onion, finely chopped
- 2 cloves garlic, minced
- 1/2 cup dry white wine
- 1/2 cup plain Greek yogurt
- 1 teaspoon Dijon mustard
- 1/4 cup grated Parmesan cheese
- 1/4 teaspoon ground black pepper
- 2 tablespoons fresh parsley, chopped

Instructions:

1. Preheat the oven to 375°F (190°C).
2. In a skillet, heat the olive oil over medium heat. Add the onion and garlic, and sauté until softened, about 3-4 minutes.
3. Add the white wine and cook for 2-3 minutes, until the liquid is reduced by half.
4. Stir in the Greek yogurt, Dijon mustard, Parmesan cheese, and black pepper. Cook for 2-3 minutes, until the sauce is thickened.
5. Add the chopped lobster meat to the skillet and mix well to coat with the sauce.
6. Transfer the mixture to a baking dish and bake for 10-12 minutes, until the top is golden brown.
7. Sprinkle with fresh parsley before serving.

Nutrition Info per Serving (Serves 2):

- Calories: 400
- Protein: 40g
- Carbohydrates: 10g
- Dietary Fiber: 1g
- Sugars: 4g
- Total Fat: 20g
- Saturated Fat: 6g
- Sodium: 450mg

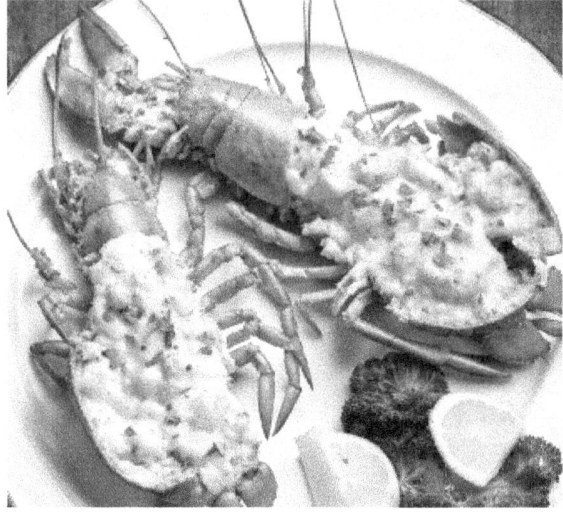

Servings: 2 Cooking Time: 20 minutes

23. Scallop and Corn Chowder

Ingredients:

- 1 pound scallops
- 2 tablespoons olive oil
- 1 onion, chopped
- 2 cloves garlic, minced
- 2 cups corn kernels (fresh or frozen)
- 2 cups low-sodium chicken broth
- 1 cup unsweetened almond milk
- 1 large potato, peeled and diced
- 1 teaspoon dried thyme
- 1/4 teaspoon ground black pepper
- 1/4 cup fresh parsley, chopped

Instructions:

1. In a large pot, heat the olive oil over medium heat. Add the chopped onion and garlic, and sauté until softened, about 3-4 minutes.
2. Add the diced potato, corn kernels, chicken broth, almond milk, thyme, and black pepper to the pot. Bring to a boil, then reduce heat and simmer for 15-20 minutes, until the potatoes are tender.
3. In a separate skillet, sear the scallops over medium-high heat for 2-3 minutes per side until golden brown and cooked through.
4. Add the seared scallops to the chowder and simmer for an additional 5 minutes.
5. Stir in the chopped parsley and serve hot.

Nutrition Info per Serving (Serves 4):

- Calories: 280
- Protein: 22g
- Carbohydrates: 32g
- Dietary Fiber: 5g
- Sugars: 5g
- Total Fat: 10g
- Saturated Fat: 1g
- Sodium: 300mg

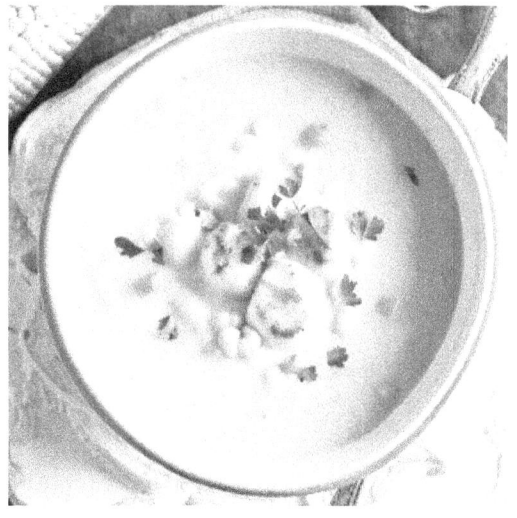

Servings: 4 Cooking Time: 30 minutes

24. Grilled Shrimp with Mango Salsa

Ingredients:

- 1 pound shrimp, peeled and deveined
- 2 tablespoons olive oil
- 1 teaspoon garlic powder
- 1/4 teaspoon ground black pepper

Mango Salsa:

- 1 ripe mango, peeled and diced
- 1/2 red bell pepper, diced
- 1/4 red onion, finely chopped
- 1/4 cup fresh cilantro, chopped
- 1 lime, juiced

Instructions:

1. Preheat the grill to medium-high heat.
2. Toss the shrimp with olive oil, garlic powder, and black pepper. Thread the shrimp onto skewers.
3. Grill the shrimp for 2-3 minutes on each side, until pink and opaque.
4. While the shrimp is grilling, prepare the mango salsa by combining the diced mango, red bell pepper, red onion, cilantro, and lime juice in a bowl. Mix well.
5. Serve the grilled shrimp topped with mango salsa.

Nutrition Info per Serving (Serves 4):

- Calories: 220
- Protein: 25g
- Carbohydrates: 12g
- Dietary Fiber: 3g
- Sugars: 8g
- Total Fat: 8g
- Saturated Fat: 1.5g
- Sodium: 320mg

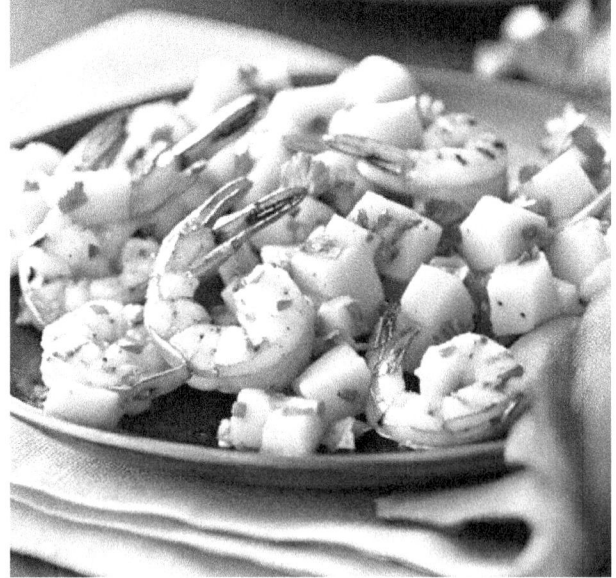

Servings: 4 Cooking Time: 15 minutes

25. Octopus Salad with Mediterranean Vegetables

Ingredients:

- 1 pound cooked octopus, sliced
- 2 tablespoons olive oil
- 1 cucumber, diced
- 1 cup cherry tomatoes, halved
- 1/4 cup red onion, thinly sliced
- 1/4 cup kalamata olives, pitted and sliced
- 1/4 cup crumbled feta cheese
- 2 tablespoons lemon juice
- 1 teaspoon dried oregano
- 1/4 teaspoon ground black pepper

Instructions:

1. In a large bowl, combine the sliced octopus, cucumber, cherry tomatoes, red onion, olives, and feta cheese.
2. In a small bowl, whisk together the olive oil, lemon juice, oregano, and black pepper.
3. Pour the dressing over the salad and toss to combine.
4. Serve immediately or refrigerate until ready to serve.

Nutrition Info per Serving (Serves 4):

- Calories: 260
- Protein: 24g
- Carbohydrates: 10g
- Dietary Fiber: 3g
- Sugars: 4g
- Total Fat: 14g
- Saturated Fat: 3g
- Sodium: 380mg

Servings: 4 Cooking Time: 15 minutes

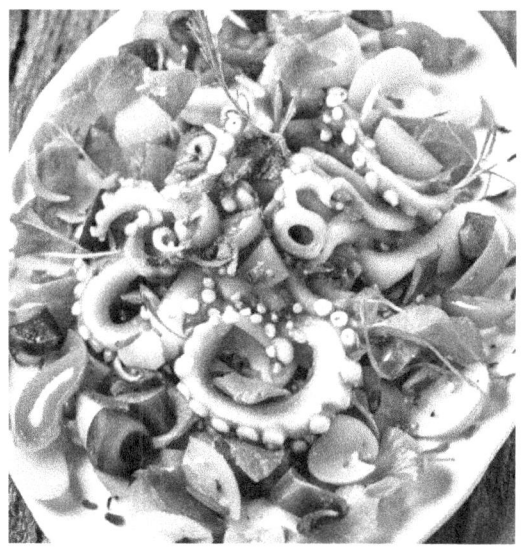

Vegetables

1. Chickpea and Spinach Salad

Ingredients:

- 1 can (15 oz) chickpeas, drained and rinsed
- 4 cups fresh spinach, chopped
- 1/2 red onion, thinly sliced
- 1/2 cup cherry tomatoes, halved
- 1/4 cup feta cheese, crumbled
- 1/4 cup chopped fresh parsley
- 2 tablespoons olive oil
- 1 tablespoon lemon juice
- 1/4 teaspoon ground black pepper

Instructions:

1. In a large bowl, combine the chickpeas, spinach, red onion, cherry tomatoes, feta cheese, and parsley.
2. In a small bowl, whisk together the olive oil, lemon juice, and black pepper.
3. Pour the dressing over the salad and toss to combine.
4. Serve immediately.

Nutrition Info per Serving (Serves 4):

- Calories: 220
- Protein: 7g
- Carbohydrates: 20g
- Dietary Fiber: 6g
- Sugars: 4g
- Total Fat: 12g
- Saturated Fat: 3g
- Sodium: 240mg

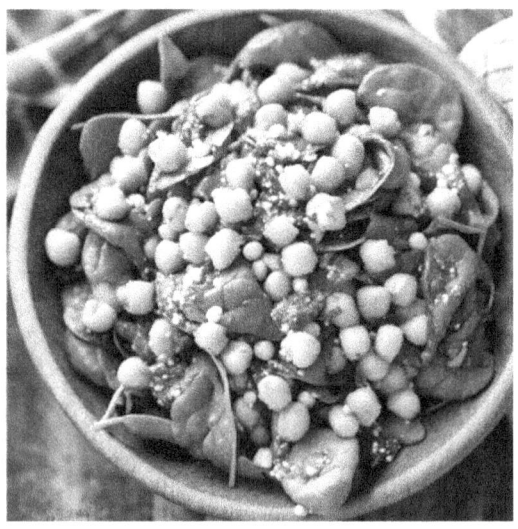

Servings: 4 Cooking Time: 10 minutes

2. Marinated Zucchini Salad

Ingredients:

- 4 medium zucchinis, thinly sliced
- 1/4 cup olive oil
- 2 tablespoons red wine vinegar
- 1 clove garlic, minced
- 1 teaspoon dried oregano
- 1/4 teaspoon ground black pepper
- 1/4 cup fresh mint leaves, chopped

Instructions:

1. In a large bowl, combine the olive oil, red wine vinegar, garlic, oregano, and black pepper.
2. Add the zucchini slices to the bowl and toss to coat.
3. Let the zucchini marinate in the refrigerator for at least 30 minutes.
4. Before serving, sprinkle with fresh mint leaves.
5. Serve chilled.

Nutrition Info per Serving (Serves 4):

- Calories: 140
- Protein: 2g
- Carbohydrates: 8g
- Dietary Fiber: 2g
- Sugars: 5g
- Total Fat: 12g
- Saturated Fat: 2g
- Sodium: 20mg

Servings: 4 Cooking Time: 40 minutes (including marinating time)

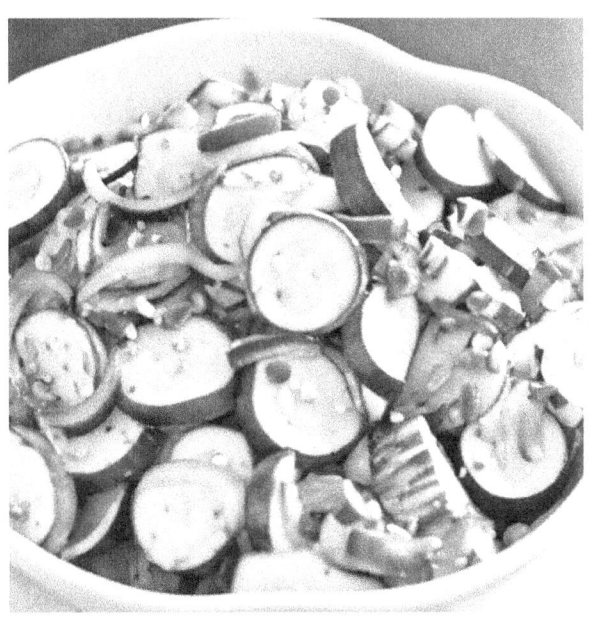

3. Greek Salad

Ingredients:

- 4 cups chopped romaine lettuce
- 1 cucumber, diced
- 1 cup cherry tomatoes, halved
- 1/4 red onion, thinly sliced
- 1/2 cup kalamata olives, pitted and halved
- 1/4 cup crumbled feta cheese
- 2 tablespoons olive oil
- 1 tablespoon red wine vinegar
- 1 teaspoon dried oregano
- 1/4 teaspoon ground black pepper

Instructions:

1. In a large bowl, combine the romaine lettuce, cucumber, cherry tomatoes, red onion, olives, and feta cheese.
2. In a small bowl, whisk together the olive oil, red wine vinegar, oregano, and black pepper.
3. Pour the dressing over the salad and toss to combine.
4. Serve immediately.

Nutrition Info per Serving (Serves 4):

- Calories: 180
- Protein: 4g
- Carbohydrates: 10g
- Dietary Fiber: 3g
- Sugars: 5g
- Total Fat: 14g
- Saturated Fat: 3g
- Sodium: 380mg

Servings: 4 Cooking Time: 10 minutes

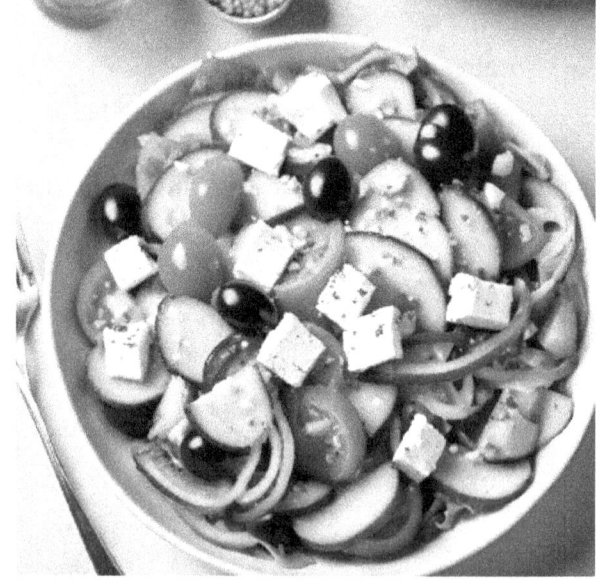

4. Avocado Tomato Salad

Ingredients:

- 2 ripe avocados, diced
- 1 cup cherry tomatoes, halved
- 1/4 red onion, finely chopped
- 1/4 cup fresh cilantro, chopped
- 1 tablespoon lime juice
- 2 tablespoons olive oil
- 1/4 teaspoon ground black pepper

Instructions:

1. In a large bowl, combine the diced avocados, cherry tomatoes, red onion, and cilantro.
2. In a small bowl, whisk together the lime juice, olive oil, and black pepper.
3. Pour the dressing over the salad and toss to combine.
4. Serve immediately.

Nutrition Info per Serving (Serves 4):

- Calories: 220
- Protein: 2g
- Carbohydrates: 12g
- Dietary Fiber: 7g
- Sugars: 2g
- Total Fat: 20g
- Saturated Fat: 3g
- Sodium: 10mg

Servings: 4 Cooking Time: 10 minutes

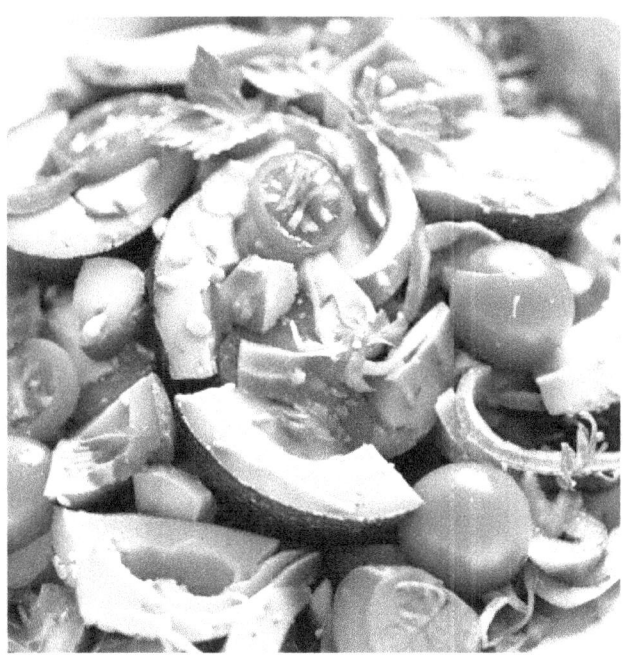

5. Spinach and Strawberry Salad

Ingredients:

- 4 cups fresh spinach, chopped
- 2 cups fresh strawberries, hulled and sliced
- 1/4 cup slivered almonds
- 1/4 cup crumbled feta cheese
- 2 tablespoons balsamic vinegar
- 1 tablespoon olive oil
- 1 teaspoon honey
- 1/4 teaspoon ground black pepper

Instructions:

1. In a large bowl, combine the spinach, strawberries, almonds, and feta cheese.
2. In a small bowl, whisk together the balsamic vinegar, olive oil, honey, and black pepper.
3. Pour the dressing over the salad and toss to combine.
4. Serve immediately.

Nutrition Info per Serving (Serves 4):

- Calories: 160
- Protein: 4g
- Carbohydrates: 13g
- Dietary Fiber: 4g
- Sugars: 8g
- Total Fat: 11g
- Saturated Fat: 2g
- Sodium: 160mg

Servings: 4 Cooking Time: 10 minutes

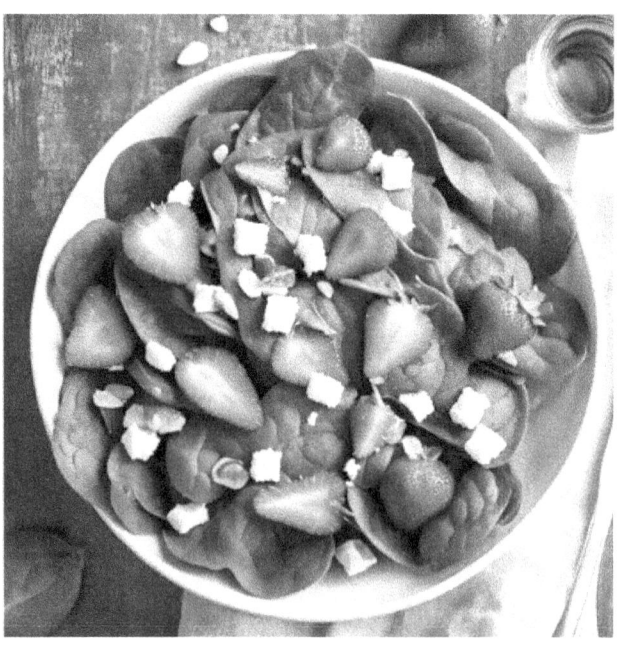

6. Vegetable Minestrone

Ingredients:

- 2 tablespoons olive oil
- 1 onion, chopped
- 2 cloves garlic, minced
- 2 carrots, diced
- 2 celery stalks, diced
- 1 zucchini, diced
- 1 yellow squash, diced
- 1 can (14.5 oz) diced tomatoes, no salt added
- 1 can (15 oz) cannellini beans, drained and rinsed
- 4 cups low-sodium vegetable broth
- 1 cup whole wheat pasta
- 1 teaspoon dried oregano
- 1 teaspoon dried basil
- 1/4 teaspoon ground black pepper
- 2 cups fresh spinach, chopped

Instructions:

1. Heat the olive oil in a large pot over medium heat. Add the onion and garlic, and sauté until softened, about 3-4 minutes.
2. Add the carrots, celery, zucchini, and yellow squash. Cook for another 5 minutes, stirring occasionally.
3. Stir in the diced tomatoes, cannellini beans, vegetable broth, oregano, basil, and black pepper. Bring to a boil.
4. Add the whole wheat pasta and reduce the heat to a simmer. Cook for 10-12 minutes, or until the pasta is tender.
5. Stir in the chopped spinach and cook for an additional 2 minutes, until wilted.
6. Serve hot.

Nutrition Info per Serving (Serves 6):

- Calories: 200
- Protein: 7g
- Carbohydrates: 33g
- Dietary Fiber: 8g
- Sugars: 7g
- Total Fat: 6g
- Saturated Fat: 1g
- Sodium: 220mg

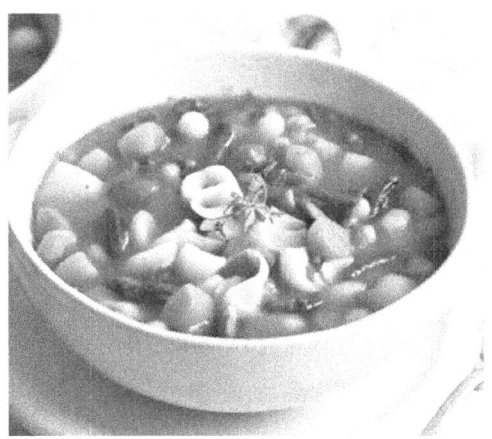

Servings: 6 Cooking Time: 30 minutes

7. Carrot Ginger Soup

Ingredients:

- 2 tablespoons olive oil
- 1 onion, chopped
- 2 cloves garlic, minced
- 1 tablespoon fresh ginger, grated
- 6 large carrots, peeled and chopped
- 4 cups low-sodium vegetable broth
- 1 teaspoon ground cumin
- 1/4 teaspoon ground black pepper
- 1/2 cup coconut milk

Instructions:

1. Heat the olive oil in a large pot over medium heat. Add the onion, garlic, and ginger, and sauté until softened, about 5 minutes.
2. Add the chopped carrots, vegetable broth, cumin, and black pepper. Bring to a boil.
3. Reduce heat and simmer for 20-25 minutes, until the carrots are tender.
4. Use an immersion blender to puree the soup until smooth. Alternatively, let the soup cool slightly and puree in batches in a blender.
5. Stir in the coconut milk and heat through.
6. Serve hot.

Nutrition Info per Serving (Serves 4):

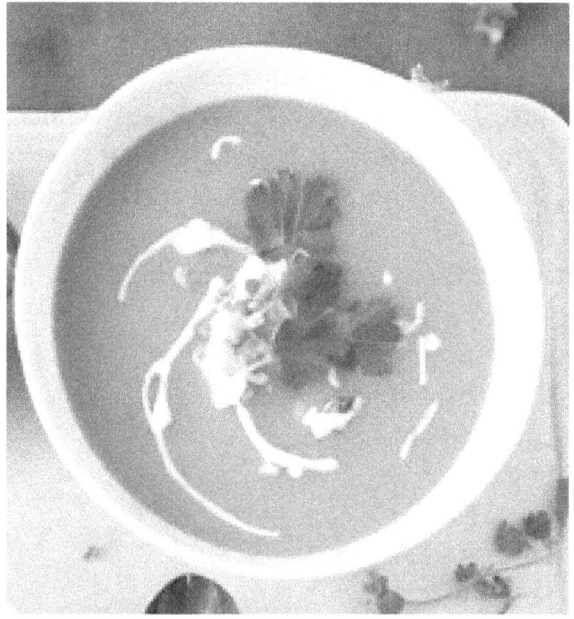

- Calories: 180
- Protein: 2g
- Carbohydrates: 22g
- Dietary Fiber: 5g
- Sugars: 10g
- Total Fat: 10g
- Saturated Fat: 6g
- Sodium: 150mg

Servings: 4 Cooking Time: 30 minutes

8. Lentil and Vegetable Stew

Ingredients:

- 2 tablespoons olive oil
- 1 onion, chopped
- 2 cloves garlic, minced
- 2 carrots, diced
- 2 celery stalks, diced
- 1 cup dried lentils, rinsed
- 1 can (14.5 oz) diced tomatoes, no salt added
- 4 cups low-sodium vegetable broth
- 1 teaspoon dried thyme
- 1 teaspoon ground cumin
- 1/4 teaspoon ground black pepper
- 2 cups chopped kale

Instructions:

1. Heat the olive oil in a large pot over medium heat. Add the onion and garlic, and sauté until softened, about 3-4 minutes.
2. Add the carrots and celery, and cook for another 5 minutes.
3. Stir in the lentils, diced tomatoes, vegetable broth, thyme, cumin, and black pepper. Bring to a boil.
4. Reduce heat and simmer for 30-35 minutes, until the lentils are tender.
5. Stir in the chopped kale and cook for an additional 5 minutes, until wilted.
6. Serve hot.

Nutrition Info per Serving (Serves 6):

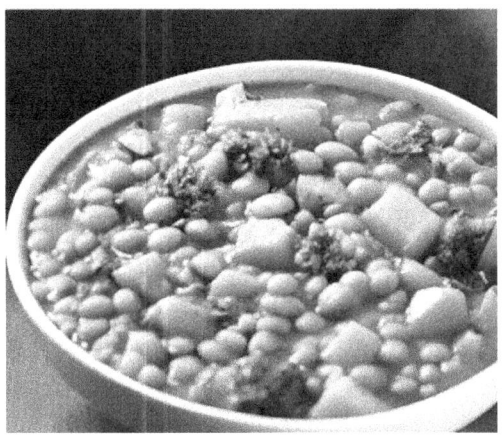

- Calories: 220
- Protein: 10g
- Carbohydrates: 35g
- Dietary Fiber: 12g
- Sugars: 8g
- Total Fat: 6g
- Saturated Fat: 1g
- Sodium: 210mg

Servings: 6 Cooking Time: 45 minutes

9. Spiced Butternut Squash Soup

Ingredients:

- 2 tablespoons olive oil
- 1 onion, chopped
- 2 cloves garlic, minced
- 1 butternut squash, peeled, seeded, and cubed
- 1 teaspoon ground cumin
- 1/2 teaspoon ground cinnamon
- 1/4 teaspoon ground black pepper
- 4 cups low-sodium vegetable broth
- 1/2 cup coconut milk

Instructions:

1. Heat the olive oil in a large pot over medium heat. Add the onion and garlic, and sauté until softened, about 3-4 minutes.
2. Add the cubed butternut squash, cumin, cinnamon, and black pepper. Cook for 5 minutes, stirring occasionally.
3. Pour in the vegetable broth and bring to a boil.
4. Reduce heat and simmer for 20-25 minutes, until the squash is tender.
5. Use an immersion blender to puree the soup until smooth. Alternatively, let the soup cool slightly and puree in batches in a blender.
6. Stir in the coconut milk and heat through.
7. Serve hot.

Nutrition Info per Serving (Serves 4):

- Calories: 200
- Protein: 3g
- Carbohydrates: 28g
- Dietary Fiber: 5g
- Sugars: 7g
- Total Fat: 10g
- Saturated Fat: 6g
- Sodium: 180mg

Servings: 4 Cooking Time: 30 minutes

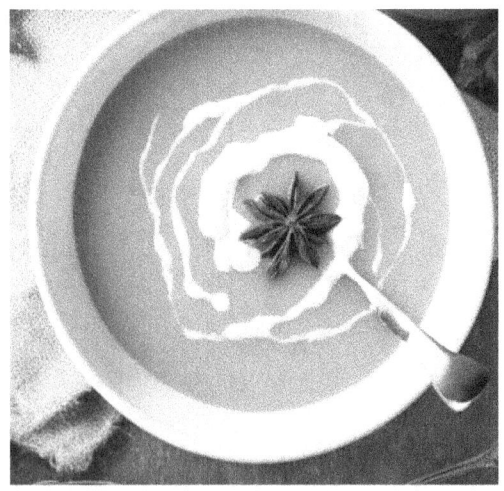

10. Sweet Potato and Black Bean Chili

Ingredients:

- 2 tablespoons olive oil
- 1 onion, chopped
- 2 cloves garlic, minced
- 2 large sweet potatoes, peeled and diced
- 1 red bell pepper, chopped
- 1 can (14.5 oz) diced tomatoes, no salt added
- 1 can (15 oz) black beans, drained and rinsed
- 1 cup low-sodium vegetable broth
- 1 tablespoon chili powder
- 1 teaspoon ground cumin
- 1/4 teaspoon ground black pepper
- 1/4 cup fresh cilantro, chopped

Instructions:

1. Heat the olive oil in a large pot over medium heat. Add the onion and garlic, and sauté until softened, about 3-4 minutes.
2. Add the diced sweet potatoes and red bell pepper, and cook for another 5 minutes.
3. Stir in the diced tomatoes, black beans, vegetable broth, chili powder, cumin, and black pepper. Bring to a boil.
4. Reduce heat and simmer for 20-25 minutes, until the sweet potatoes are tender.
5. Stir in the chopped cilantro before serving.
6. Serve hot.

Nutrition Info per Serving (Serves 6):

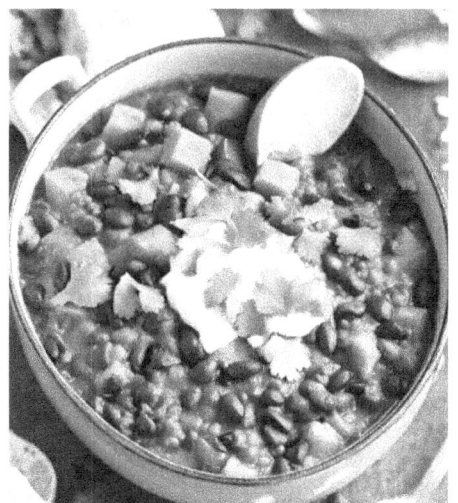

- Calories: 250
- Protein: 6g
- Carbohydrates: 45g
- Dietary Fiber: 10g
- Sugars: 11g
- Total Fat: 6g
- Saturated Fat: 1g
- Sodium: 200mg

Servings: 6 Cooking Time: 35 minutes

11. Cream of Asparagus Soup

Ingredients:

- 2 tablespoons olive oil
- 1 onion, chopped
- 2 cloves garlic, minced
- 2 pounds asparagus, trimmed and cut into 1-inch pieces
- 4 cups low-sodium vegetable broth
- 1 cup unsweetened almond milk
- 1 teaspoon dried thyme
- 1/4 teaspoon ground black pepper
- 1 tablespoon lemon juice

Instructions:

1. Heat the olive oil in a large pot over medium heat. Add the onion and garlic, and sauté until softened, about 3-4 minutes.
2. Add the asparagus and cook for another 5 minutes, stirring occasionally.
3. Pour in the vegetable broth and add the dried thyme and black pepper. Bring to a boil.
4. Reduce heat and simmer for 15-20 minutes, until the asparagus is tender.
5. Use an immersion blender to puree the soup until smooth. Alternatively, let the soup cool slightly and puree in batches in a blender.
6. Stir in the almond milk and lemon juice, and heat through.
7. Serve hot.

Nutrition Info per Serving (Serves 4):

- Calories: 160
- Protein: 4g
- Carbohydrates: 15g
- Dietary Fiber: 4g
- Sugars: 5g
- Total Fat: 9g
- Saturated Fat: 1g
- Sodium: 190mg

Servings: 4 Cooking Time: 30 minutes

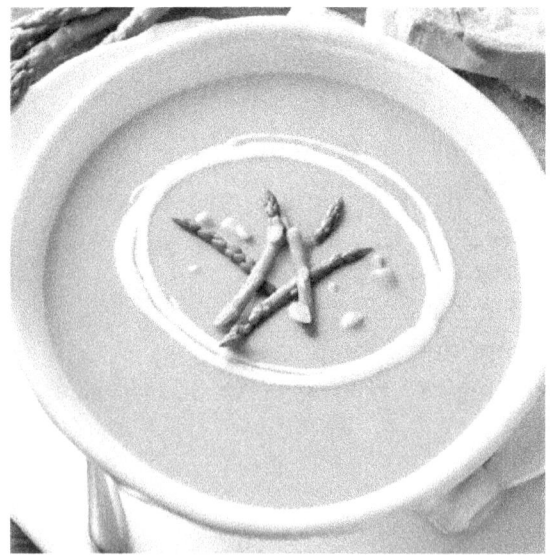

12. Stuffed Bell Peppers

Ingredients:

- 4 large bell peppers, tops cut off and seeds removed
- 1 cup cooked quinoa
- 1 can (15 oz) black beans, drained and rinsed
- 1 cup corn kernels (fresh or frozen)
- 1/2 cup diced tomatoes
- 1/2 cup chopped onion
- 2 cloves garlic, minced
- 2 tablespoons olive oil
- 1 teaspoon ground cumin
- 1/4 teaspoon ground black pepper
- 1/2 cup shredded mozzarella cheese, part-skim

Instructions:

1. Preheat the oven to 375°F (190°C).
2. In a large skillet, heat the olive oil over medium heat. Add the onion and garlic, and sauté until softened, about 3-4 minutes.
3. Stir in the cooked quinoa, black beans, corn, diced tomatoes, cumin, and black pepper. Cook for another 5 minutes, stirring occasionally.
4. Remove from heat and stir in the shredded mozzarella cheese.
5. Stuff the bell peppers with the quinoa mixture and place them in a baking dish.
6. Cover the dish with aluminum foil and bake for 25-30 minutes, until the peppers are tender.
7. Serve hot.

Nutrition Info per Serving (Serves 4):

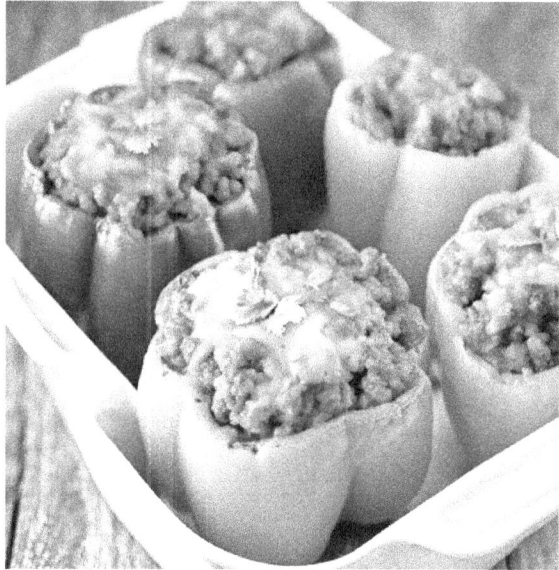

- Calories: 260
- Protein: 10g
- Carbohydrates: 34g
- Dietary Fiber: 9g
- Sugars: 10g
- Total Fat: 10g
- Saturated Fat: 3g
- Sodium: 200mg

Servings: 4 Cooking Time: 40 minutes

13. Eggplant Parmesan

Ingredients:

- 2 large eggplants, sliced into 1/4-inch rounds
- 1/4 cup olive oil
- 1 cup whole wheat breadcrumbs
- 1/2 cup grated Parmesan cheese
- 2 cups marinara sauce, no salt added
- 1 cup shredded mozzarella cheese, part-skim
- 1 teaspoon dried basil
- 1/4 teaspoon ground black pepper

Instructions:

1. Preheat the oven to 375°F (190°C).
2. In a shallow bowl, combine the breadcrumbs, Parmesan cheese, dried basil, and black pepper.
3. Brush the eggplant slices with olive oil and coat each slice with the breadcrumb mixture.
4. Place the breaded eggplant slices on a baking sheet and bake for 20-25 minutes, until golden brown.
5. Spread 1 cup of marinara sauce in the bottom of a baking dish. Layer half of the eggplant slices over the sauce.
6. Spread another cup of marinara sauce over the eggplant slices and sprinkle with half of the shredded mozzarella cheese.
7. Repeat the layers with the remaining eggplant slices, marinara sauce, and mozzarella cheese.
8. Bake for 25-30 minutes, until the cheese is melted and bubbly.
9. Serve hot.

Nutrition Info per Serving (Serves 4):

- Calories: 300
- Protein: 14g
- Carbohydrates: 34g
- Dietary Fiber: 10g
- Sugars: 15g
- Total Fat: 14g
- Saturated Fat: 4.5g
- Sodium: 360mg

Servings: 4 Cooking Time: 55 minutes

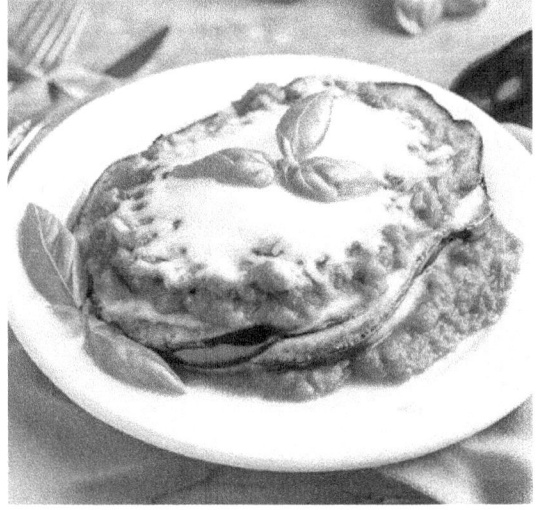

14. Zucchini Noodles with Pesto

Ingredients:

- 4 medium zucchinis, spiralized into noodles
- 1/2 cup basil pesto (store-bought or homemade)
- 1 tablespoon olive oil
- 1/4 cup cherry tomatoes, halved
- 1/4 cup grated Parmesan cheese
- 1/4 teaspoon ground black pepper

Instructions:

1. Heat the olive oil in a large skillet over medium heat. Add the zucchini noodles and cook for 2-3 minutes, until just tender.
2. Remove from heat and toss the zucchini noodles with the basil pesto until well coated.
3. Add the cherry tomatoes and toss gently to combine.
4. Sprinkle with grated Parmesan cheese and ground black pepper.
5. Serve immediately.

Nutrition Info per Serving (Serves 4):

- Calories: 180
- Protein: 6g
- Carbohydrates: 8g
- Dietary Fiber: 3g
- Sugars: 5g
- Total Fat: 14g
- Saturated Fat: 3g
- Sodium: 190mg

Servings: 4 Cooking Time: 10 minutes

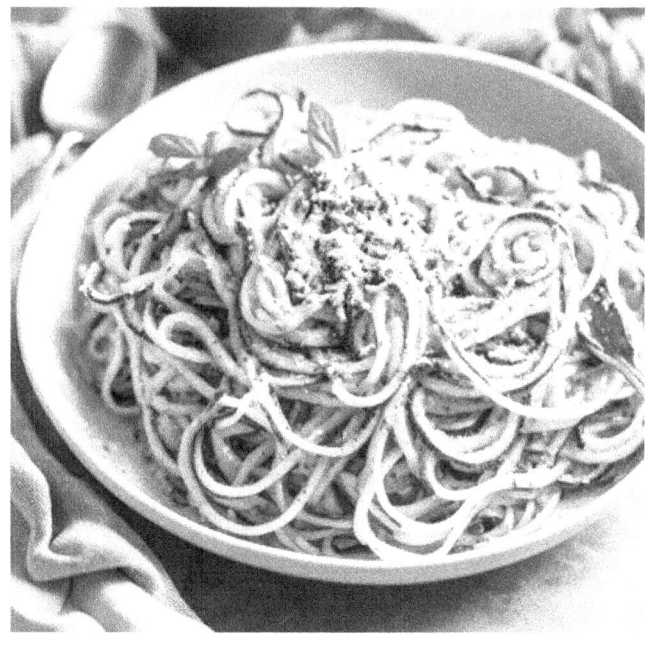

15. Mushroom Risotto

Ingredients:

- 2 tablespoons olive oil
- 1 onion, chopped
- 2 cloves garlic, minced
- 1 pound mushrooms, sliced
- 1 cup arborio rice
- 1/2 cup dry white wine (optional)
- 4 cups low-sodium vegetable broth, warmed
- 1/2 cup grated Parmesan cheese
- 1/4 cup chopped fresh parsley
- 1/4 teaspoon ground black pepper

Instructions:

1. Heat the olive oil in a large skillet over medium heat. Add the onion and garlic, and sauté until softened, about 3-4 minutes.
2. Add the sliced mushrooms and cook until they release their juices and become tender, about 5-7 minutes.
3. Stir in the arborio rice and cook for 2-3 minutes until the rice is lightly toasted.
4. If using, add the white wine and cook until it is mostly absorbed, about 2 minutes.
5. Begin adding the warmed vegetable broth, one ladleful at a time, stirring frequently and allowing the liquid to be absorbed before adding more. Continue this process until the rice is creamy and tender, about 20-25 minutes.
6. Stir in the grated Parmesan cheese, chopped parsley, and ground black pepper.
7. Serve hot.

Nutrition Info per Serving (Serves 4):

- Calories: 300
- Protein: 9g
- Carbohydrates: 44g
- Dietary Fiber: 4g
- Sugars: 5g
- Total Fat: 10g
- Saturated Fat: 2.5g
- Sodium: 250mg

Servings: 4 Cooking Time: 40 minutes

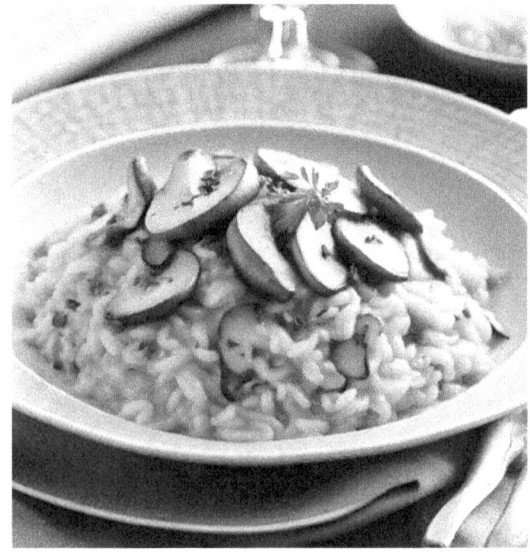

16. Spaghetti Squash with Marinara

Ingredients:

- 1 large spaghetti squash
- 2 tablespoons olive oil
- 1 onion, chopped
- 2 cloves garlic, minced
- 1 can (28 oz) crushed tomatoes, no salt added
- 1 teaspoon dried basil
- 1 teaspoon dried oregano
- 1/4 teaspoon ground black pepper
- 1/4 cup grated Parmesan cheese
- 1/4 cup fresh basil, chopped

Instructions:

1. Preheat the oven to 400°F (200°C).
2. Cut the spaghetti squash in half lengthwise and scoop out the seeds. Drizzle with 1 tablespoon of olive oil and place cut-side down on a baking sheet. Roast for 40-45 minutes, or until the squash is tender and easily pierced with a fork.
3. While the squash is roasting, heat the remaining olive oil in a large skillet over medium heat. Add the chopped onion and garlic, and sauté until softened, about 5 minutes.
4. Stir in the crushed tomatoes, dried basil, oregano, and black pepper. Simmer for 20 minutes, stirring occasionally.
5. Once the squash is done, use a fork to scrape out the spaghetti-like strands into a serving bowl.
6. Pour the marinara sauce over the spaghetti squash and toss to combine.
7. Sprinkle with grated Parmesan cheese and chopped fresh basil before serving.

Nutrition Info per Serving (Serves 4):

- Calories: 220
- Protein: 5g
- Carbohydrates: 30g
- Dietary Fiber: 7g
- Sugars: 12g
- Total Fat: 10g
- Saturated Fat: 2g
- Sodium: 200mg

Servings: 4 Cooking Time: 50 minutes

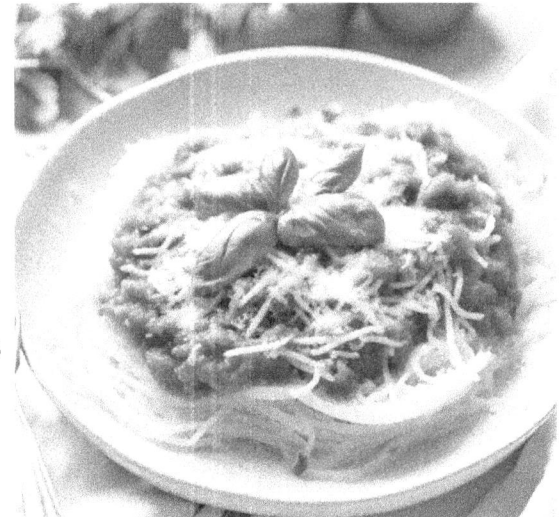

17. Garlic Roasted Brussels Sprouts

Ingredients:

- 1 1/2 pounds Brussels sprouts, trimmed and halved
- 3 tablespoons olive oil
- 3 cloves garlic, minced
- 1/4 teaspoon ground black pepper
- 1/4 cup grated Parmesan cheese

Instructions:

1. Preheat the oven to 400°F (200°C).
2. In a large bowl, toss the Brussels sprouts with olive oil, minced garlic, and black pepper.
3. Spread the Brussels sprouts in a single layer on a baking sheet.
4. Roast for 20-25 minutes, stirring halfway through, until the sprouts are golden brown and tender.
5. Remove from the oven and sprinkle with grated Parmesan cheese.
6. Serve immediately.

Nutrition Info per Serving (Serves 4):

- Calories: 180
- Protein: 5g
- Carbohydrates: 14g
- Dietary Fiber: 6g
- Sugars: 3g
- Total Fat: 13g
- Saturated Fat: 2.5g
- Sodium: 180mg

Servings: 4 Cooking Time: 30 minutes

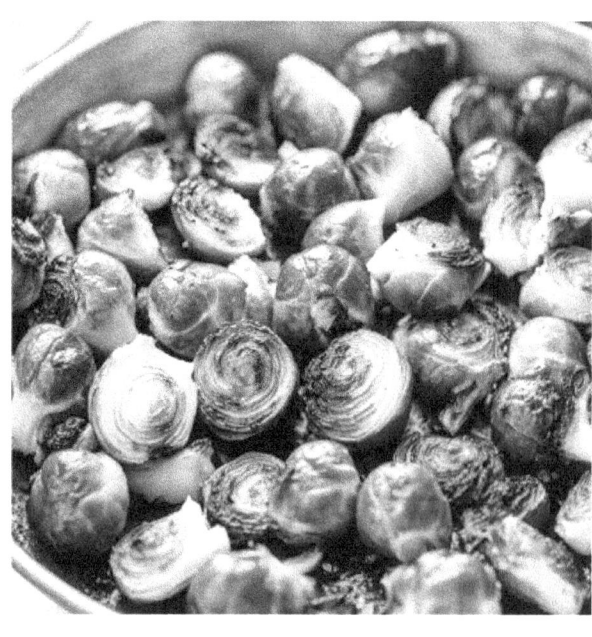

18. Sweet Potato Wedges

Ingredients:
- 3 large sweet potatoes, cut into wedges
- 2 tablespoons olive oil
- 1 teaspoon ground cumin
- 1/2 teaspoon paprika
- 1/4 teaspoon ground black pepper

Instructions:
1. Preheat the oven to 425°F (220°C).
2. In a large bowl, toss the sweet potato wedges with olive oil, ground cumin, paprika, and black pepper.
3. Arrange the sweet potato wedges in a single layer on a baking sheet.
4. Roast for 25-30 minutes, turning halfway through, until the wedges are golden brown and tender.
5. Serve immediately.

Nutrition Info per Serving (Serves 4):
- Calories: 200
- Protein: 3g
- Carbohydrates: 36g
- Dietary Fiber: 6g
- Sugars: 9g
- Total Fat: 7g
- Saturated Fat: 1g
- Sodium: 80mg

Servings: 4 Cooking Time: 30 minutes

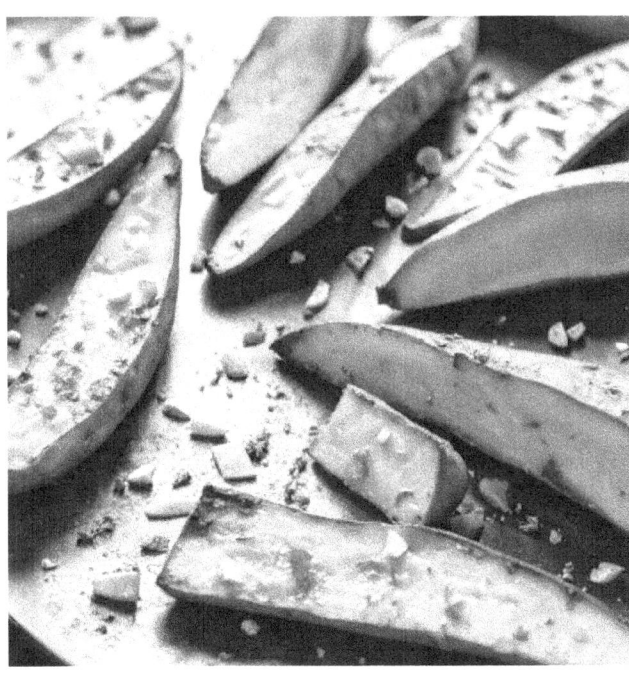

19. Green Beans Almondine

Ingredients:

- 1 pound green beans, trimmed
- 2 tablespoons olive oil
- 3 cloves garlic, minced
- 1/4 cup sliced almonds
- 1 tablespoon lemon juice
- 1/4 teaspoon ground black pepper

Instructions:

1. Bring a large pot of water to a boil. Add the green beans and blanch for 3-4 minutes, until bright green and just tender. Drain and set aside.
2. In a large skillet, heat the olive oil over medium heat. Add the minced garlic and sliced almonds, and sauté for 2-3 minutes until the almonds are golden brown and the garlic is fragrant.
3. Add the blanched green beans to the skillet and toss to combine.
4. Drizzle with lemon juice and sprinkle with black pepper.
5. Serve immediately.

Nutrition Info per Serving (Serves 4):

- Calories: 130
- Protein: 3g
- Carbohydrates: 8g
- Dietary Fiber: 4g
- Sugars: 2g
- Total Fat: 10g
- Saturated Fat: 1.5g
- Sodium: 40mg

Servings: 4 Cooking Time: 15 minutes

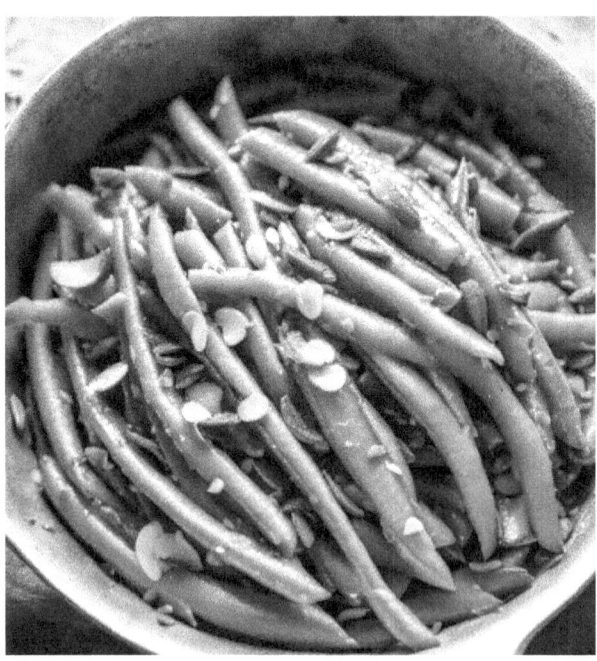

20. Balsamic Glazed Carrots

Ingredients:

- 1 pound carrots, peeled and cut into sticks
- 2 tablespoons olive oil
- 2 tablespoons balsamic vinegar
- 1 tablespoon honey
- 1/4 teaspoon ground black pepper

Instructions:

1. Preheat the oven to 400°F (200°C).
2. In a large bowl, toss the carrot sticks with olive oil, balsamic vinegar, honey, and black pepper.
3. Arrange the carrots in a single layer on a baking sheet.
4. Roast for 20-25 minutes, stirring halfway through, until the carrots are tender and caramelized.
5. Serve immediately.

Nutrition Info per Serving (Serves 4):

- Calories: 140
- Protein: 1g
- Carbohydrates: 16g
- Dietary Fiber: 4g
- Sugars: 10g
- Total Fat: 8g
- Saturated Fat: 1g
- Sodium: 60mg

Servings: 4 Cooking Time: 25 minutes

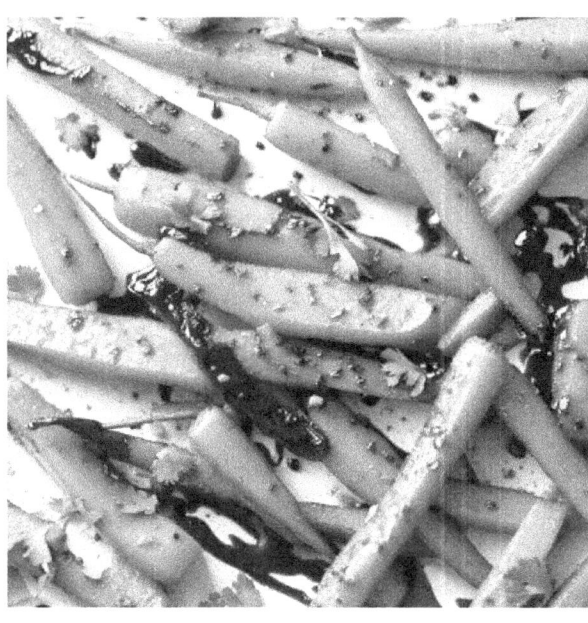

21. Sauteed Spinach with Garlic

Ingredients:

- 2 tablespoons olive oil
- 4 cloves garlic, minced
- 1 pound fresh spinach, washed and trimmed
- 1/4 teaspoon ground black pepper
- 1 tablespoon lemon juice

Instructions:

1. Heat the olive oil in a large skillet over medium heat.
2. Add the minced garlic and sauté for about 1 minute until fragrant.
3. Add the spinach in batches, stirring constantly until wilted, about 3-4 minutes.
4. Sprinkle with ground black pepper and lemon juice, then toss to combine.
5. Serve immediately.

Nutrition Info per Serving (Serves 4):

- Calories: 90
- Protein: 3g
- Carbohydrates: 7g
- Dietary Fiber: 4g
- Sugars: 1g
- Total Fat: 7g
- Saturated Fat: 1g
- Sodium: 60mg

Servings: 4 Cooking Time: 10 minutes

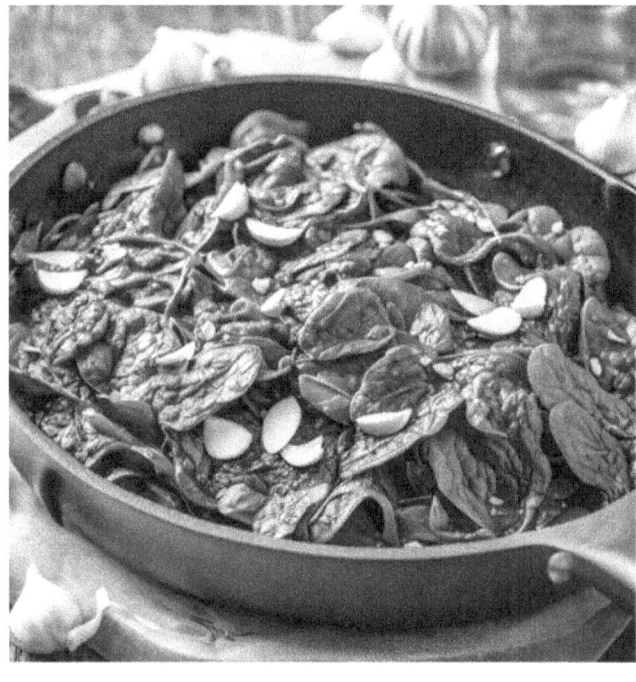

22. Roasted Beet Chips

Ingredients:

- 4 medium beets, peeled and thinly sliced
- 2 tablespoons olive oil
- 1/4 teaspoon ground black pepper

Instructions:

1. Preheat the oven to 375°F (190°C).
2. Toss the beet slices with olive oil and ground black pepper.
3. Arrange the beet slices in a single layer on a baking sheet lined with parchment paper.
4. Roast for 30-35 minutes, turning halfway through, until the beet chips are crispy.
5. Let cool slightly before serving.

Nutrition Info per Serving (Serves 4):

- Calories: 110
- Protein: 2g
- Carbohydrates: 13g
- Dietary Fiber: 4g
- Sugars: 9g
- Total Fat: 7g
- Saturated Fat: 1g
- Sodium: 60mg

Servings: 4 Cooking Time: 35 minutes

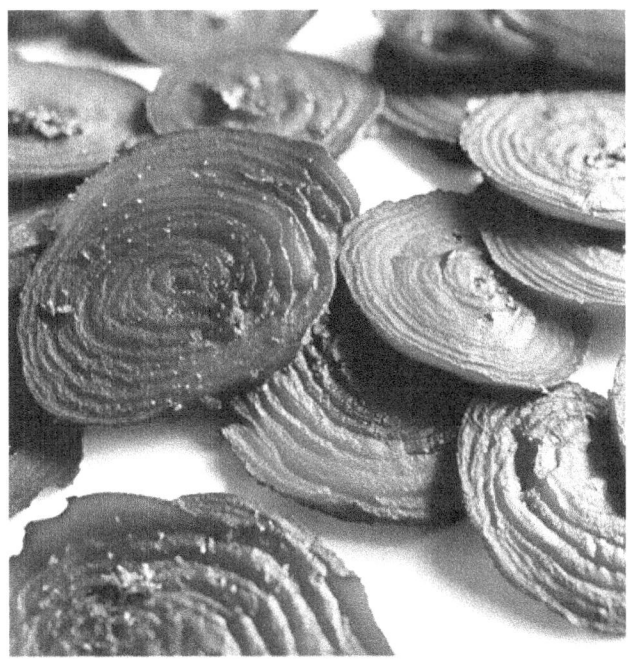

23. Baked Apple Slices with Cinnamon

Ingredients:

- 4 large apples, cored and thinly sliced
- 2 tablespoons coconut oil, melted
- 1 teaspoon ground cinnamon
- 1 tablespoon honey

Instructions:

1. Preheat the oven to 350°F (175°C).
2. Toss the apple slices with melted coconut oil, ground cinnamon, and honey.
3. Arrange the apple slices in a single layer on a baking sheet lined with parchment paper.
4. Bake for 20-25 minutes, until the apples are tender and slightly caramelized.
5. Serve warm.

Nutrition Info per Serving (Serves 4):

- Calories: 160
- Protein: 1g
- Carbohydrates: 29g
- Dietary Fiber: 5g
- Sugars: 22g
- Total Fat: 6g
- Saturated Fat: 4g
- Sodium: 0mg

Servings: 4 Cooking Time: 25 minutes

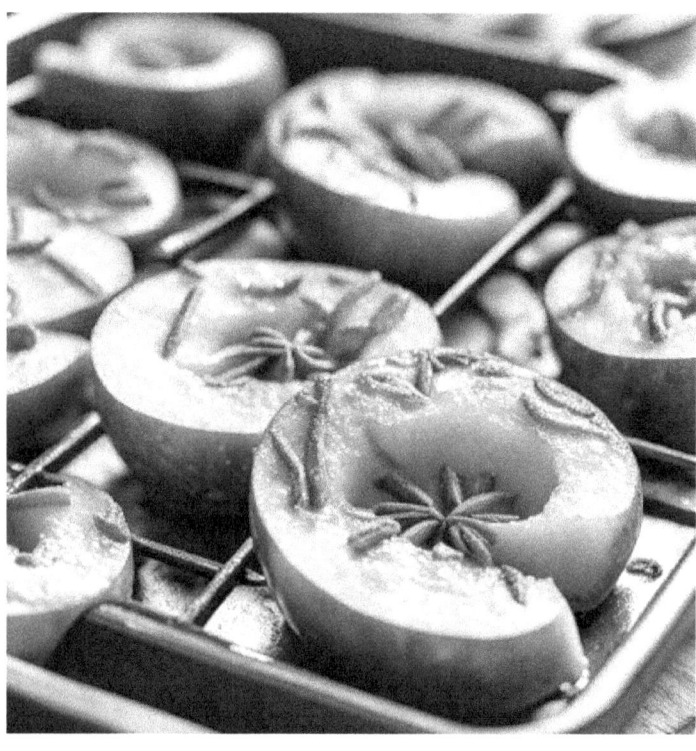

24. Pea and Mint Dip

Ingredients:

- 2 cups frozen peas, thawed
- 1/4 cup fresh mint leaves
- 2 tablespoons olive oil
- 1 clove garlic, minced
- 1 tablespoon lemon juice
- 1/4 teaspoon ground black pepper

Instructions:

1. In a food processor, combine the thawed peas, mint leaves, olive oil, minced garlic, lemon juice, and black pepper.
2. Blend until smooth, scraping down the sides as needed.
3. Transfer to a serving bowl and serve with whole grain crackers or vegetable sticks.

Nutrition Info per Serving (Serves 4):

- Calories: 110
- Protein: 4g
- Carbohydrates: 15g
- Dietary Fiber: 5g
- Sugars: 6g
- Total Fat: 5g
- Saturated Fat: 1g
- Sodium: 20mg

Servings: 4 Cooking Time: 10 minutes

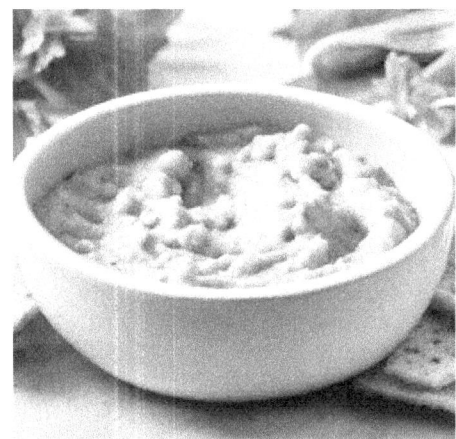

25. Baked Zucchini Fries

Ingredients:

- 3 medium zucchinis, cut into fries
- 1/2 cup whole wheat breadcrumbs
- 1/4 cup grated Parmesan cheese
- 1 teaspoon garlic powder
- 1 teaspoon dried oregano
- 2 large eggs, beaten
- 1/4 teaspoon ground black pepper

Instructions:

1. Preheat the oven to 425°F (220°C).
2. In a shallow bowl, combine the breadcrumbs, Parmesan cheese, garlic powder, oregano, and black pepper.
3. Dip the zucchini fries into the beaten eggs, then coat with the breadcrumb mixture.
4. Arrange the zucchini fries in a single layer on a baking sheet lined with parchment paper.
5. Bake for 20-25 minutes, turning halfway through, until the zucchini fries are golden brown and crispy.
6. Serve immediately.

Nutrition Info per Serving (Serves 4):

- Calories: 150
- Protein: 7g
- Carbohydrates: 16g
- Dietary Fiber: 3g
- Sugars: 3g
- Total Fat: 7g
- Saturated Fat: 2g
- Sodium: 200mg

Servings: 4 Cooking Time: 25 minutes

10-WEEK MEAL PLAN

Week 1
Monday
- Breakfast: Oatmeal with Blueberries
- Lunch: Chickpea and Spinach Salad
- Dinner: Grilled Salmon with Dill Yogurt Sauce, Garlic Roasted Brussels Sprouts

Tuesday
- Breakfast: Spinach and Feta Omelette
- Lunch: Greek Salad
- Dinner: Lemon Herb Roasted Chicken, Sweet Potato Wedges

Wednesday
- Breakfast: Greek Yogurt Parfait
- Lunch: Marinated Zucchini Salad
- Dinner: Baked Cod with Lemon and Capers, Green Beans Almondine

Thursday
- Breakfast: Whole Grain Pancakes
- Lunch: Avocado Tomato Salad
- Dinner: Chicken and Spinach Soup, Balsamic Glazed Carrots

Friday
- Breakfast: Quinoa Porridge
- Lunch: Vegetable Minestrone
- Dinner: Turmeric Chicken Stir-Fry, Steamed Brown Rice

Saturday
- Breakfast: Turkey Sausage and Veggie Hash
- Lunch: Sweet Potato and Black Bean Chili
- Dinner: Herb-Baked Tilapia, Roasted Beet Chips

Sunday
- Breakfast: Mushroom and Spinach Frittata
- Lunch: Lentil and Vegetable Stew
- Dinner: Chicken Piccata with Capers, Sauteed Spinach with Garlic

Week 2
Monday
- Breakfast: Almond Butter Banana Toast
- Lunch: Spinach and Strawberry Salad
- Dinner: Tandoori Chicken, Cauliflower Rice

Tuesday
- Breakfast: Kale and Tomato Quiche
- Lunch: Stuffed Bell Peppers
- Dinner: Sesame Chicken and Broccoli, Quinoa

Wednesday
- Breakfast: Berry and Walnut Oatmeal
- Lunch: Spiced Butternut Squash Soup
- Dinner: Balsamic Chicken Salad, Zucchini Noodles with Pesto

Thursday
- Breakfast: Vegetable Muffins
- Lunch: Turkey and Cranberry Salad
- Dinner: Grilled Mackerel with Salsa Verde, Baked Zucchini Fries

Friday
- Breakfast: Pumpkin Spice Smoothie
- Lunch: Green Beans Almondine
- Dinner: Moroccan Chicken Stew, Couscous

Saturday
- Breakfast: Broccoli and Cheese Omelette
- Lunch: Pea and Mint Dip with Whole Grain Crackers
- Dinner: Curried Shrimp and Quinoa Salad, Steamed Asparagus

Sunday
- Breakfast: Sweet Potato and Kale Bowl
- Lunch: Spaghetti Squash with Marinara
- Dinner: Flounder with Parsley and Garlic, Roasted Carrots

Week 3

Monday
- Breakfast: Apple Cinnamon Steel-Cut Oats
- Lunch: Tomato Basil Soup with Whole Grain Bread
- Dinner: Greek Chicken Skewers, Mixed Green Salad

Tuesday
- Breakfast: Muesli with Skim Milk
- Lunch: Sweet Potato and Black Bean Chili
- Dinner: Turkey Meatballs in Tomato Basil Sauce, Steamed Broccoli

Wednesday
- Breakfast: Mixed Berry Compote with Yogurt
- Lunch: Mushroom Risotto
- Dinner: Salmon Patties with Lemon Aioli, Steamed Green Beans

Thursday
- Breakfast: Pistachio and Peach Yogurt
- Lunch: Balsamic Glazed Carrots
- Dinner: Mediterranean Chicken Wrap, Marinated Zucchini Salad

Friday
- Breakfast: Spinach and Mushroom Toast
- Lunch: Beet and Berry Juice
- Dinner: Chicken and Barley Soup, Roasted Beet Chips

Saturday
- Breakfast: Buckwheat Porridge
- Lunch: Avocado Tomato Salad
- Dinner: Grilled Shrimp with Mango Salsa, Sweet Potato Wedges

Sunday
- Breakfast: Egg and Avocado Salad
- Lunch: Roasted Beet Chips
- Dinner: Stuffed Turkey Breast with Spinach and Walnuts, Sauteed Spinach with Garlic

Week 4

Monday
- Breakfast: Peanut Butter Oatmeal
- Lunch: Zucchini Noodles with Pesto
- Dinner: Herb Roasted Turkey Thighs, Garlic Roasted Brussels Sprouts

Tuesday
- Breakfast: Veggie and Herb Cream Cheese Spread on Whole Grain Toast
- Lunch: Lentil and Vegetable Stew
- Dinner: Spaghetti Squash with Marinara, Green Beans Almondine

Wednesday
- Breakfast: Beet and Berry Juice
- Lunch: Baked Apple Slices with Cinnamon
- Dinner: Baked Sardines with Herbs, Sweet Potato Wedges

Thursday
- Breakfast: Spinach and Citrus Salad
- Lunch: Sweet Potato and Kale Bowl
- Dinner: Fish Stew with Tomatoes and Olives, Roasted Carrots

Friday
- Breakfast: Pumpkin Spice Smoothie
- Lunch: Vegetable Minestrone
- Dinner: Turkey and Spinach Meatloaf, Balsamic Glazed Carrots

Saturday
- Breakfast: Broccoli and Cheese Omelette
- Lunch: Chickpea and Spinach Salad
- Dinner: Lobster Thermidor, Garlic Roasted Brussels Sprouts

Sunday
- Breakfast: Sweet Potato and Kale Bowl
- Lunch: Marinated Zucchini Salad
- Dinner: Roasted Trout with Fennel, Sauteed Spinach with Garlic

Week 5

Monday
- Breakfast: Muesli with Skim Milk
- Lunch: Greek Salad
- Dinner: Pan-Seared Trout with Almonds, Green Beans Almondine

Tuesday
- Breakfast: Mixed Berry Compote with Yogurt
- Lunch: Spiced Butternut Squash Soup
- Dinner: Chicken Cauliflower Fried Rice, Steamed Asparagus

Wednesday
- Breakfast: Pistachio and Peach Yogurt
- Lunch: Sweet Potato and Black Bean Chili
- Dinner: Octopus Salad with Mediterranean Vegetables, Baked Zucchini Fries

Thursday
- Breakfast: Spinach and Mushroom Toast
- Lunch: Avocado Tomato Salad
- Dinner: Scallop and Corn Chowder, Steamed Green Beans

Friday
- Breakfast: Buckwheat Porridge
- Lunch: Pea and Mint Dip with Whole Grain Crackers
- Dinner: Turkey Picadillo, Sauteed Spinach with Garlic

Saturday
- Breakfast: Egg and Avocado Salad
- Lunch: Spaghetti Squash with Marinara
- Dinner: Italian Turkey and Zucchini Skillet, Roasted Beet Chips

Sunday
- Breakfast: Peanut Butter Oatmeal
- Lunch: Baked Apple Slices with Cinnamon
- Dinner: Shrimp Caesar Salad, Garlic Roasted Brussels Sprouts

Week 6

Monday
- Breakfast: Sauteed Spinach with Garlic
- Lunch: Marinated Zucchini Salad
- Dinner: Grilled Calamari with Olive Oil and Lemon, Balsamic Glazed Carrots

Tuesday
- Breakfast: Vegetable Muffins
- Lunch: Pea and Mint Dip with Vegetable Sticks
- Dinner: Turkey Stew with Root Vegetables, Roasted Beet Chips

Wednesday
- Breakfast: Pumpkin Spice Smoothie
- Lunch: Spaghetti Squash with Marinara
- Dinner: Herb-Baked Tilapia, Sweet Potato Wedges

Thursday
- Breakfast: Broccoli and Cheese Omelette
- Lunch: Avocado Tomato Salad
- Dinner: Grilled Shrimp with Mango Salsa, Steamed Green Beans

Friday
- Breakfast: Sweet Potato and Kale Bowl
- Lunch: Chickpea and Spinach Salad
- Dinner: Moroccan Chicken Stew, Couscous

Saturday
- Breakfast: Apple Cinnamon Steel-Cut Oats
- Lunch: Lentil and Vegetable Stew
- Dinner: Flounder with Parsley and Garlic, Garlic Roasted Brussels Sprouts

Sunday
- Breakfast: Muesli with Skim Milk
- Lunch: Baked Apple Slices with Cinnamon
- Dinner: Chicken Piccata with Capers, Sauteed Spinach with Garlic

Week 7

Monday
- Breakfast: Mixed Berry Compote with Yogurt
- Lunch: Sweet Potato and Black Bean Chili
- Dinner: Turkey Meatballs in Tomato Basil Sauce, Roasted Carrots

Tuesday
- Breakfast: Pistachio and Peach Yogurt
- Lunch: Greek Salad
- Dinner: Pan-Seared Trout with Almonds, Green Beans Almondine

Wednesday
- Breakfast: Spinach and Mushroom Toast
- Lunch: Tomato Basil Soup with Whole Grain Bread
- Dinner: Balsamic Chicken Salad, Steamed Asparagus

Thursday
- Breakfast: Buckwheat Porridge
- Lunch: Spiced Butternut Squash Soup
- Dinner: Grilled Mackerel with Salsa Verde, Baked Zucchini Fries

Friday
- Breakfast: Egg and Avocado Salad
- Lunch: Pea and Mint Dip with Whole Grain Crackers
- Dinner: Curried Shrimp and Quinoa Salad, Steamed Green Beans

Saturday
- Breakfast: Peanut Butter Oatmeal
- Lunch: Marinated Zucchini Salad
- Dinner: Herb Roasted Turkey Thighs, Sweet Potato Wedges

Sunday
- Breakfast: Veggie and Herb Cream Cheese Spread on Whole Grain Toast
- Lunch: Lentil and Vegetable Stew
- Dinner: Grilled Salmon with Dill Yogurt Sauce, Sauteed Spinach with Garlic

Week 8

Monday
- Breakfast: Sauteed Spinach with Garlic
- Lunch: Baked Apple Slices with Cinnamon
- Dinner: Baked Sardines with Herbs, Garlic Roasted Brussels Sprouts

Tuesday
- Breakfast: Vegetable Muffins
- Lunch: Avocado Tomato Salad
- Dinner: Chicken and Barley Soup, Sweet Potato Wedges

Wednesday
- Breakfast: Pumpkin Spice Smoothie
- Lunch: Pea and Mint Dip with Vegetable Sticks
- Dinner: Pan-Seared Trout with Almonds, Balsamic Glazed Carrots

Thursday
- Breakfast: Broccoli and Cheese Omelette
- Lunch: Spiced Butternut Squash Soup
- Dinner: Moroccan Chicken Stew, Couscous

Friday
- Breakfast: Sweet Potato and Kale Bowl
- Lunch: Chickpea and Spinach Salad
- Dinner: Herb-Baked Tilapia, Green Beans Almondine

Saturday
- Breakfast: Apple Cinnamon Steel-Cut Oats
- Lunch: Lentil and Vegetable Stew
- Dinner: Grilled Calamari with Olive Oil and Lemon, Roasted Beet Chips

Sunday
- Breakfast: Muesli with Skim Milk
- Lunch: Greek Salad
- Dinner: Turkey Stew with Root Vegetables, Garlic Roasted Brussels Sprouts

Week 9

Monday
- Breakfast: Mixed Berry Compote with Yogurt
- Lunch: Sweet Potato and Black Bean Chili
- Dinner: Tandoori Chicken, Cauliflower Rice

Tuesday
- Breakfast: Pistachio and Peach Yogurt
- Lunch: Spaghetti Squash with Marinara
- Dinner: Grilled Shrimp with Mango Salsa, Balsamic Glazed Carrots

Wednesday
- Breakfast: Spinach and Mushroom Toast
- Lunch: Tomato Basil Soup with Whole Grain Bread
- Dinner: Moroccan Chicken Stew, Steamed Green Beans

Thursday
- Breakfast: Buckwheat Porridge
- Lunch: Spiced Butternut Squash Soup
- Dinner: Herb Roasted Turkey Thighs, Sweet Potato Wedges

Friday
- Breakfast: Egg and Avocado Salad
- Lunch: Pea and Mint Dip with Whole Grain Crackers
- Dinner: Flounder with Parsley and Garlic, Garlic Roasted Brussels Sprouts

Saturday
- Breakfast: Peanut Butter Oatmeal
- Lunch: Baked Apple Slices with Cinnamon
- Dinner: Scallop and Corn Chowder, Steamed Green Beans

Sunday
- Breakfast: Veggie and Herb Cream Cheese Spread on Whole Grain Toast
- Lunch: Avocado Tomato Salad
- Dinner: Grilled Salmon with Dill Yogurt Sauce, Balsamic Glazed Carrots

Week 10

Monday
- Breakfast: Sauteed Spinach with Garlic
- Lunch: Marinated Zucchini Salad
- Dinner: Pan-Seared Trout with Almonds, Sweet Potato Wedges

Tuesday
- Breakfast: Vegetable Muffins
- Lunch: Greek Salad
- Dinner: Curried Shrimp and Quinoa Salad, Garlic Roasted Brussels Sprouts

Wednesday
- Breakfast: Pumpkin Spice Smoothie
- Lunch: Pea and Mint Dip with Vegetable Sticks
- Dinner: Turkey Stew with Root Vegetables, Green Beans Almondine

Thursday
- Breakfast: Broccoli and Cheese Omelette
- Lunch: Spiced Butternut Squash Soup
- Dinner: Herb-Baked Tilapia, Roasted Carrots

Friday
- Breakfast: Sweet Potato and Kale Bowl
- Lunch: Chickpea and Spinach Salad
- Dinner: Grilled Calamari with Olive Oil and Lemon, Balsamic Glazed Carrots

Saturday
- Breakfast: Apple Cinnamon Steel-Cut Oats
- Lunch: Sweet Potato and Black Bean Chili
- Dinner: Herb Roasted Turkey Thighs, Garlic Roasted Brussels Sprouts

Sunday
- Breakfast: Muesli with Skim Milk
- Lunch: Lentil and Vegetable Stew
- Dinner: Grilled Mackerel with Salsa Verde, Steamed Green Beans

WEEKLY MEAL PLANNER + WORKBOOK

	BREAKFAST	LUNCH	DINNER	SNACKS
MONDAY				
TUESDAY				
WEDNESDAY				
THURSDAY				
FRIDAY				
SATURDAY				
SUNDAY				

Reflect on your current eating habits. What are some of your favorite foods and meals?

....

....

....

....

....

....

WEEKLY MEAL PLANNER + WORKBOOK

	BREAKFAST	LUNCH	DINNER	SNACKS
MONDAY				
TUESDAY				
WEDNESDAY				
THURSDAY				
FRIDAY				
SATURDAY				
SUNDAY				

What inspired you to consider starting the MIND diet?

WEEKLY MEAL PLANNER + WORKBOOK

	BREAKFAST	LUNCH	DINNER	SNACKS
MONDAY				
TUESDAY				
WEDNESDAY				
THURSDAY				
FRIDAY				
SATURDAY				
SUNDAY				

List three foods you currently enjoy that are already part of the MIND diet. How can you incorporate them into your meals more regularly?

....

....

....

....

....

....

WEEKLY MEAL PLANNER + WORKBOOK

	BREAKFAST	LUNCH	DINNER	SNACKS
MONDAY				
TUESDAY				
WEDNESDAY				
THURSDAY				
FRIDAY				
SATURDAY				
SUNDAY				

Consider your grocery shopping routine. How can you adjust it to include more MIND diet-friendly foods?

....

....

....

....

....

....

WEEKLY MEAL PLANNER + WORKBOOK

	BREAKFAST	LUNCH	DINNER	SNACKS
MONDAY				
TUESDAY				
WEDNESDAY				
THURSDAY				
FRIDAY				
SATURDAY				
SUNDAY				

What challenges or concerns do you anticipate when starting the MIND diet? How do you plan to overcome them?

....

....

....

....

....

....

WEEKLY MEAL PLANNER + WORKBOOK

	BREAKFAST	LUNCH	DINNER	SNACKS
MONDAY				
TUESDAY				
WEDNESDAY				
THURSDAY				
FRIDAY				
SATURDAY				
SUNDAY				

Identify three new MIND diet foods or ingredients you're willing to incorporate into your meals. What interests you about these choices?

....

....

....

....

....

....

WEEKLY MEAL PLANNER + WORKBOOK

	BREAKFAST	LUNCH	DINNER	SNACKS
MONDAY				
TUESDAY				
WEDNESDAY				
THURSDAY				
FRIDAY				
SATURDAY				
SUNDAY				

How do you plan to manage social gatherings or dining out while following the MIND diet?

....

....

....

....

....

....

WEEKLY MEAL PLANNER + WORKBOOK

	BREAKFAST	LUNCH	DINNER	SNACKS
MONDAY				
TUESDAY				
WEDNESDAY				
THURSDAY				
FRIDAY				
SATURDAY				
SUNDAY				

Reflect on your current cooking skills. What new recipes or cooking techniques are you interested in trying as part of the MIND diet?

....

....

....

....

....

....

WEEKLY MEAL PLANNER + WORKBOOK

	BREAKFAST	LUNCH	DINNER	SNACKS
MONDAY				
TUESDAY				
WEDNESDAY				
THURSDAY				
FRIDAY				
SATURDAY				
SUNDAY				

Consider your support system. How can family members or friends assist you in maintaining the MIND diet?

....

....

....

....

....

....

WEEKLY MEAL PLANNER + WORKBOOK

	BREAKFAST	LUNCH	DINNER	SNACKS
MONDAY				
TUESDAY				
WEDNESDAY				
THURSDAY				
FRIDAY				
SATURDAY				
SUNDAY				

Reflect on any dietary restrictions or health concerns you have. How can the MIND diet support your overall health and well-being?

....

....

....

....

....

....

WEEKLY MEAL PLANNER + WORKBOOK

	BREAKFAST	LUNCH	DINNER	SNACKS
MONDAY				
TUESDAY				
WEDNESDAY				
THURSDAY				
FRIDAY				
SATURDAY				
SUNDAY				

What are your goals for starting the MIND diet? How will you measure your progress towards these goals?

....

....

....

....

....

....

WEEKLY MEAL PLANNER + WORKBOOK

	BREAKFAST	LUNCH	DINNER	SNACKS
MONDAY				
TUESDAY				
WEDNESDAY				
THURSDAY				
FRIDAY				
SATURDAY				
SUNDAY				

What role does physical activity play in your daily routine? How can you integrate exercise with your dietary goals on the MIND diet?

....

....

....

....

....

....

WEEKLY MEAL PLANNER + WORKBOOK

	BREAKFAST	LUNCH	DINNER	SNACKS
MONDAY				
TUESDAY				
WEDNESDAY				
THURSDAY				
FRIDAY				
SATURDAY				
SUNDAY				

Reflect on any changes in taste preferences you've experienced over the years. How can you adapt your meals to fit these preferences while on the MIND diet?

....

....

....

....

....

....

WEEKLY MEAL PLANNER + WORKBOOK

	BREAKFAST	LUNCH	DINNER	SNACKS
MONDAY				
TUESDAY				
WEDNESDAY				
THURSDAY				
FRIDAY				
SATURDAY				
SUNDAY				

What emotional or psychological strategies can you employ to stay motivated and committed to the MIND diet?

....

....

....

....

....

....

Scan the QR code below to get a surprise bonus!

www.ingramcontent.com/pod-product-compliance
Lightning Source LLC
Chambersburg PA
CBHW082235220526
45479CB00005B/1243